# RETHINKING DRINKING

## The Influence That Everyone's Under

CRAIG NOBLE

2nd 20, LLC
Fort Lauderdale, Florida

*Rethinking Drinking: The Influence That Everyone's Under*

Copyright © 2020 Craig Noble

Published by 2nd 20, LLC
Fort Lauderdale, Florida

Cover and Interior Design by Imagine! Studios
www.ArtsImagine.com

Cover Images: Scrudje/Bigstock.com; iStock.com/Nastco

ISBN: 978-1-7348275-0-7 (hardback)
ISBN: 978-1-7348275-1-4 (e-book)

Library of Congress Control Number: 2020938722

First Printing: June 2020

*For Ty*

# CONTENTS

This is your last chance. After this,
there is no turning back. You take the
*blue* pill . . . and believe whatever
you want to believe. You take the *red*
pill . . . and I show you how deep the
rabbit hole goes. Remember: all I'm
offering is the truth. Nothing more.

Morpheus
*The Matrix*, 1999

# Introduction

I grew up with alcohol consumed all around me. Mostly beer, and mostly by the men in my family. I also remember a few Saturday afternoons when my mother would have a vodka with grapefruit juice fresh from the tree next door while she and my Dad were sitting outside visiting with our neighbors. Otherwise, my Mother liked to drink hot tea while reading or socializing. I also grew up recognizing the beer brand all the adult men drank around me—the one in the TV ads that showed it being pulled in a regal carriage by majestic horses. All of that TV and real life familiarity made me ask my Dad to let me sip his beer now and then, which he did. But most of all, my experience with alcohol growing up was as a sort of routine background constant for socializing adults, and I never thought much of it—until my own son started asking me about it.

His questions about the taste of the different alcohol types and brands started when he was a preteen, which were prompted when he saw an alcohol commercial on TV or a billboard on the highway. However, by this time in my life, my own relationship with alcohol had gone from social to habit to compulsion to dependence to addiction to abstinence, and yet it still didn't make sense to me. So, I thought it best to parent his questions by just answering about the taste of alcohol, avoiding talking about the attractive glamour of alcohol ads, and downplaying the attractive normalcy of people drinking alcohol. All that was going fine until one night, when my son was high school-aged, his reaction after a knock at our door made me want to rethink the maybe-too-brief explanations I was giving him about alcohol.

*Rethinking Drinking* is a story about our common awareness about alcohol—both conscious and subconscious. It's also a story about the super-genius of alcohol marketing. I'm a huge fan of business and marketing, and this journey to understand myself and others also led me to see that the eyes-wide-open-but-blind-consumer-loyalty achieved by the alcohol industry is absolutely-astoundingly-impressive.

If you go back and read the table of contents again, you'll see that I laid out this book in a linear progression. It starts with what happened with my neighbor as the impetus for writing this book, then moves along sort of a dot-connecting continuum of increasingly honest awareness about the effect alcohol has on all of us, and finally arrives at the reason we're all under the influence of it. Lastly, I share how I explained it all to my teenage son.

There are far too many alcohol messes that we can avoid with a little more awareness and conversation about its slick marketing and slippery effects.

Oh, and the reason I laid out this book with illustrations, common quotes, and with each chapter condensed to two facing pages is to make it fun and easy for everyone to read and talk about—even those who don't usually like to read, and even those who received it as a gift and decide to read a page or two after stumbling home drunk.

If you're reading this book as an adult, whether to better understand yourself or someone you love, you'll soon understand that it's not your parents (or your friends or the alcohol companies or the celebrity pitch people) that are to blame for whatever relationship you have with alcohol. If you're reading this book as a teenager, get ready for a wild ride of awareness, because chances are that what you've learned so far about alcohol is the world that's been pulled over your eyes to get you ready to start buying more alcohol for more occasions when you turn 21 too.

*CRAIG NOBLE*
*May 2020*

# LORENZO

Knock-Knock-Knock-Knock

All Good 'Round Here—Right?

Found Him Wandering Downtown

A Little More Is Gonna Happen

Call Duration: 7 Seconds

Not The First Time

Wakeup Slap

. . . everyone knows a Lorenzo

# Knock-Knock-Knock-Knock

I'm cooking dinner.

My son is doing trigonometry homework, texting on his phone, and watching something on TV.

It's just us in the house. It's quiet inside and dark outside, so the knock at the front screen porch door startles both of us.

As I move from the kitchen to the front of the house, I see him on the step outside the screen porch. Dark blue pants and sleeves, pistol on his hip, badge on his chest, smile on his face.

*Hi, Fort Lauderdale Police.*

I don't reply yet. I'm even more startled now, because there's no reason for the police to just stop by. We don't live in that kind of neighborhood and we don't live that kind of life.

*Do you live here?*

I'm ready to answer now, but I resist the urge to give him a smart-ass reply.

Most of my experience with cops walking up to me to say Hi, is limited to the couple times I've been pulled over for rolling through stop signs, driving through lights that turned red too fast, or driving 44 like everyone else even though the posted speed limit is 35. I haven't done things that might cause the police to want to find me at home since I was a teenager. And since my teenage son doesn't have a Bad Boy Itch that he has to scratch, I'm certain the cop isn't at my door for anything either of us had done. So my slight annoyance turns into curiosity.

*Yes, I live here. Can I help you?*

*Do you know your neighbor?*

*Sort of.*

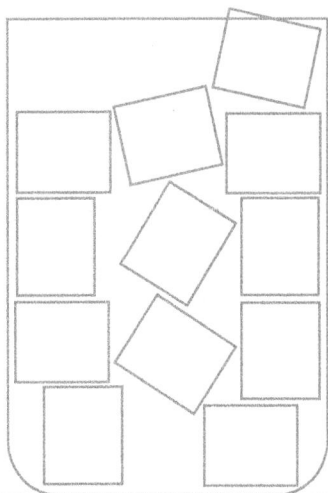

# All Good 'Round Here—Right?

I answered *Sort of*, because Lorenzo and Camilla are new neighbors. They had just moved in a month or so ago. And except for a brief but friendly introduction with Lorenzo when we each happened to be putting our trash cans out for pickup at the same time last week, I know very little about them.

They're both in their early 30s, from Brazil, and they both speak better Portuguese than English. He works most nights in a high-end restaurant, and she comes and goes throughout the day because of her job at a nearby import-export services company. They're recently married for the first time, pregnant with their first child, they have two dogs and they are first-time homeowners. They don't mind that they paid a record amount for the house and spent more money improving it before moving in, because they believe the neighborhood values are on the rise due to all of the other renovations going on around us.

So, all good news for me as the homeowner next door—right?

A smart, career-driven, family-focused young couple next door that cares for their appreciating home value probably means quiet neighbors in a well-maintained house—right?

I shouldn't pay any attention to the fact that for the month or so before I finally called out to say *Hello* to Lorenzo, or that since that exchange, I've barely seen either of them. I should also let it go that neither looks up when they are outside, which only seems to be long enough to take the trash out and then go back inside . . . or come and go in their cars and then go back inside. I also never see them walk their dogs, and they always keep their window shades closed.

Aw geez, never mind all that stuff—right?

He's probably been busy inside putting baby furniture together all day . . . her pregnancy probably makes her sensitive to daylight . . . he probably walks the dogs when he gets home from his night job, and the only reason I probably don't see them very often is because I'm busy doing my thing too. Everyone's happy and healthy—right?

In fact, I should feel like I hit the jackpot with my new neighbors. Maybe we'll get to know each other and have a TV sitcom kind of neighborly friendship. Barbeques together in the backyard . . . watch the kids play together in the front yard . . . meet each other's families when they visit, and keep an eye on the other's homes when on vacation.

So I'm not sure what the cop wants, or what he means when he asks if I know my neighbor, because it's alllll good 'round here—right?

# Found Him Wandering Downtown

*D*o you know his name?

*Yes. His name is Lorenzo.*

*Okay. Good. Do you know anything else about him? He says he and his wife just bought the house next door, just moved in, and that she's pregnant or she just had a baby, or something like that.*

*Oh, yes, all of that is true. And, yes, he told me when I met him last week that his wife is pregnant with their first baby.*

*Okay. Good. We just wanted to make sure he lives where he says he does before we let him out of the car.*

My thoughts turn from curious to stunned.

The cop looks down and away. He's thinking about whether to tell me what's going on or just say *Thanks* and walk back to his police car.

He decides to tell me.

*Well. We found him wandering around downtown. He's had a lot to drink today. Lost his phone, lost his keys, lost his wallet, doesn't remember where he parked, and his wife is not home.*

My mouth falls open. I thought I knew this guy. I can't speak.

The cop gives me a professional smile and nod.

*Have a nice evening.*

I'm still standing inside the closed screen door. I watch the cop calmly turn and walk down my driveway into the street toward his car that I can hear idling in front of Lorenzo's immaculately maintained front yard.

I can't see anything. It's too dark. I hear a car door open and close. Then I hear the cop's voice again.

*I don't know what you're gonna do.*

Lorenzo must have been asking the police officer who was kind enough to give him a ride home what he should do next. But I could only hear the cop's voice.

*Sit on your front porch. Climb the fence. Sit in your backyard. I don't know.*

I hear another car door open and close. Then I hear the police car pull away.

I feel my son push up against me from behind. He must have been hanging back inside the house listening to what the cop and I were saying, then got closer once he knew the cop stepped away.

*What's going on, Dad?*

I turn and back him up, and we both step back into the house.

*I'll tell you in a minute. This isn't over yet.*

# A Little More Is Gonna Happen

My son's expression hints that he's not liking what's going on, so I try to calm him down.

*Just gimme a minute. Everything's okay. It's just that there's gonna be a little more that's gonna happen. Then I'll be able to explain all of it to you.*

My answer seems good enough. He walks over to stand in front of the TV, which is on but muted. I guess he turned the sound off so he could hear the cop and I talk at the front door a few minutes earlier.

The kitchen timer beeps.

I walk over to turn the oven heat from *Bake* to *Warm*. I know what's coming next. But I don't know how long it's gonna take to arrive or how long it's gonna last.

BANG-RATTLE-BANG-RATTLE-BANG-RATTLE

*Craaaaaig?*

My son looks up at me from his semi-focus on the TV.

*It's okay. That's Lorenzo at the screen door. I'm going to talk to him. I'm not going to leave the house. I'm not going to let him in.*

He nods but doesn't move, because although he's heard my story about meeting Lorenzo and hearing about our great but private new neighbors, he's never heard anyone call his Dad's name with such a shaky long drawl.

I round the corner to the still-open front door, and see Lorenzo standing outside the screen porch. Blue jeans, bright white polo shirt, clean white sneakers, dim look on his face.

*Hey Lorenzo.*

Lorenzo tilts his head as he's looking in my direction, presses his mouth into a half-smile, raises his eyebrows and lifts his arms from his side, palms up.

With those four simple movements, he lets me know that he drank too much, needs help, and wants to borrow my phone to call someone.

But I ask anyway.

*What's up?*

His words are quieter and more choppy now, like six verbal bursts.

*Craig-can-I-borrow-your-phone?*

*Sure. Stay here. I'll get it for you and be right back.*

In one fluid motion, I turn, step and grab my phone from the table inside the front door, select the dial function, step back to open the screen door and hand it to Lorenzo.

In a series of slow motions, Lorenzo reaches out for my phone, manages a firm grip around it, pulls it back toward him, stutter-pecks his other index finger ten times on the dial screen, and raises it to his ear—all while balancing his slightly swaying stance.

Although my phone is not on speaker, I can hear his wife's voice answer.

*Hello?*

# Call Duration: 7 Seconds

After taking a shallow breath to steady his voice, Lorenzo replies something into the phone in Portuguese.

I don't speak Portuguese, but it sounds to me like he only says one word.

I'm leaning against the open screen door jamb.

Lorenzo is slightly swaying and looking at the ground as he holds my phone to his ear. He's not speaking, and I don't hear anything from Camilla through my phone.

I feel a little weird keeping such a close eye on what seems like a private kind of a call between my neighbor and his wife. But if he falls, I wanna catch him. One, because I don't want Lorenzo to hurt himself. Two, because I don't want him to drop my phone.

Then, following what seems like forever-silence, the strangest thing happens.

Lorenzo moves my phone from his ear so he can see the screen. Then he reaches out to hand it back to me. And without saying anything or looking up from the ground, he balances a slow turn and carefully chooses his steps down my driveway into the darkness.

I look at my phone. Call ended. Call duration 7 seconds.

Then I realize the reason I didn't hear Lorenzo or his wife talking.

She had hung up on him.

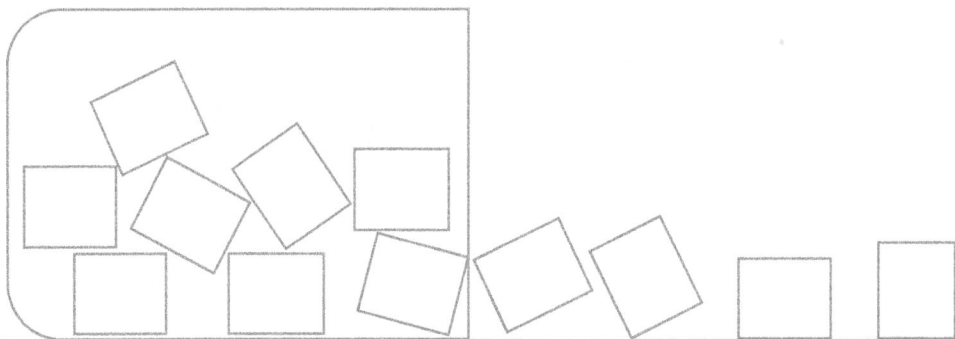

# Not The First Time

---

reach to close the screen door, and I feel my son push up against me again from behind.

*Dad. What is going on?*

We both step back into the house.

*I'm closing the front door. That's enough visitors for us tonight.*

*Yeah, close the door. What was all that?*

My son's voice and body language tell me he's still a little scared and confused, and I sense he's also getting anxious.

Deep breath. Long exhale. I answer in the most reassuring way I can.

*Lorenzo went out tonight. He drank too much, lost his keys, wallet, phone and car, and was wandering around downtown. The police must have seen him and decided to pick him up and bring him home. And since Lorenzo also lost his identification, the police knocked on our door to ask us if he lives next door before they dropped him off.*

I can tell my son understands my answer, but he doesn't like it.

*Then why did Lorenzo come knock on our door after the police left? What did he want?*

*Lorenzo's wife is not home to let him in. And since he lost his phone, he asked to borrow mine to call her.*

My son's voice then starts cramping with frustration and wanting to understand.

*So she's gonna come home and let him in?*

*I don't know what they're going to do. But I don't want to be in the middle of it. That's why I closed the door.*

*Huh?*

When Lorenzo handed my phone back to me after he called his wife, I could see on the screen that the reason I didn't hear them speaking to each other is because as soon as she heard his voice, she hung up on him.

My son is shocked.

*But he can't get in his house without her. Why did she hang up on him?*

My reply is gonna be a guess, but I feel pretty good about it being close to the truth of the matter. One, because I have been in this situation before. Two, because I have seen friends in this situation before. So I answer him.

*Because my guess is this isn't the first time Camilla has gotten that kind of drunken call for help from Lorenzo.*

The next thing that happens catches me by complete surprise.

# Wakeup Slap

**I**DIOT!

My son is angry and yelling and walking around the living room.

*Idiot! IDIOT!* **IDIOT!**

Now I'm shocked. But still calm. I manage to squeeze my question in between his bursts.

*Why is he an Idiot?*

My son is not calm, and he isn't confused anymore. He is clear and he is very frustrated about what he has just unexpectedly learned about Lorenzo.

*Because he just got married, just bought a house, and he's just about to have a baby!*

I still wasn't following his extreme reaction.

*Yes. But how does all that make him an idiot?*

He looks past me at the TV and points at the screen. In that moment, a beer commercial is on.

*Watch the bottom of the screen at the end of the commercial!*

I turn and look. The sound is still off, but we both watch the commercial. It's a group of young people on a beach smiling and laughing and each holding a beer bottle and appearing to be celebrating something. Then the commercial ends with the sweaty labeled bottle on the screen, and the small but prominently displayed words below: Drink Responsibly.

*See Dad, everybody knows how it works. You just gotta drink responsibly!*

My shock turns into intrigue as he continues to explain his adamant teenage understanding of how to drink alcohol.

*The only people that don't drink responsibly are the idiots in internet videos that drink too much and then do stupid things that happen to get caught on camera.*

*So you're saying Lorenzo is an idiot because . . . ?*

*Because he's got lots of reasons to party, but to drink so much that he lost all of his stuff, and his car, and the police had to bring him home, and he's locked out of his house, he must be STUPID!*

His answer feels like a wakeup slap in the face. Could it be that we are both right?

I can barely manage the words out of my mouth to agree with his clear and correct, although limited, understanding about what had just happened.

*Oh.*

# ONE STORY, SIX TRUTHS

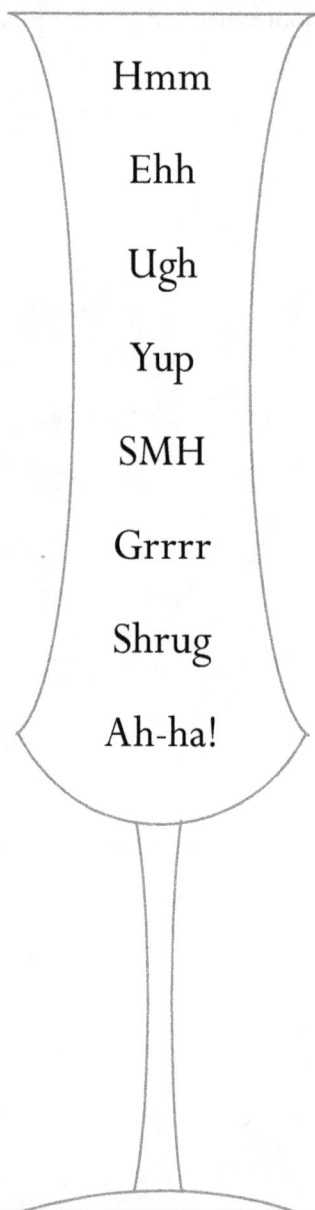

Hmm

Ehh

Ugh

Yup

SMH

Grrrr

Shrug

Ah-ha!

. . . but only one of us was drinking

# Hmm

The more I thought about what happened that night, the more fascinated I became.

I mean, if I hadn't experienced my teenage son's reaction, I would have just seen the evening's events as unfortunate but infrequent, then forgot all about it.

And I would have still believed my new neighbor was a nice guy, but also one that maybe needed some tough love from his wife, so he wouldn't make another mess, and then forgot about what was maybe going on with them too.

I realized that the five people involved that night each had a different reaction to the same experience.

And interestingly, not only did each of us believe we were crystal-clear-correct about our read on the situation, but also, only one of us was drinking. One event, five people, but so many different truths.

Hmm.

Let's start with the cop.

# Ehh

Everything about the cop's demeanor and delivery revealed his unspoken belief about the situation he encountered that night and how he chose to handle it: *Whatever.*

Since the cop's job is to protect and serve, when he sees a drunk wandering around our fancy downtown, he probably has three options. One, tell him to move along. Two, arrest him. Three, under very special circumstances, help him.

My guess about the reason the cop chose to give Lorenzo a ride home is based on a number of factors that added up in Lorenzo's favor.

First, when the cop encountered Lorenzo stumbling around like a vagrant, he also saw styled hair, shaved face, expensive clothes and new sneakers. So he probably decided to engage in a little conversation before taking action, because Lorenzo's clean-cut appearance did not at all match his destitute-level of drunken behavior.

Then, when the cop learned that Lorenzo was a nice-guy-type-of-drunk, and therefore not a threat to himself or anyone else, that's when he probably decided Lorenzo didn't need to be arrested.

And, when the cop learned Lorenzo had lost his phone and wallet, he knew Lorenzo couldn't call or pay for a ride.

Finally, when the cop learned that Lorenzo and his pregnant wife had just bought a home nearby, I think that's when the cop decided to help a good guy that maybe just made some bad choices that day.

Just my guess. But I have experience with this stuff.

It could have easily gone another way for Lorenzo that night, but he caught a break, because the cop's truth was: *Ehh, I see this all the time.*

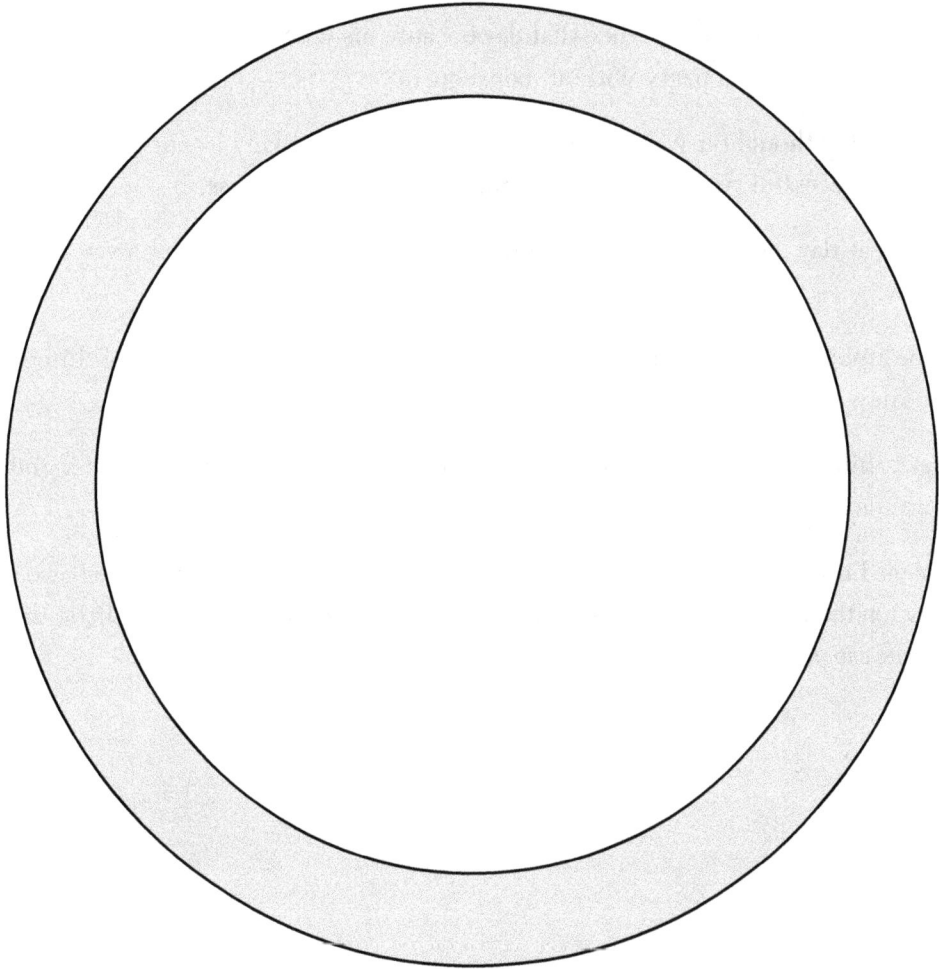

# Ugh

My experienced guess about Lorenzo's belief that evening was clear to me from his reaction: *Unlucky.*

It was like he decided to roll the dice that day because his wife was out of town and he really wanted to win a personal party without consequences.

And he probably thought it was a good bet, because he had likely learned what to do from his previous successful runs and failed attempts when on a hall pass.

However, that day, he underestimated something. What it was that got away from him, I don't know.

Maybe the amount he drank, maybe what he drank, maybe a combination of things. I don't think he knew either.

But what I think Lorenzo and I would agree about is that he planned to drink and have a have a nice day—not drink and upset his wife.

So although Lorenzo looked to me like he believed he was responsible for what happened and sorry for the mess he made, his bottom-line truth also seemed to be a little displaced: *Ugh, my wife caught me making a drinking mess again.*

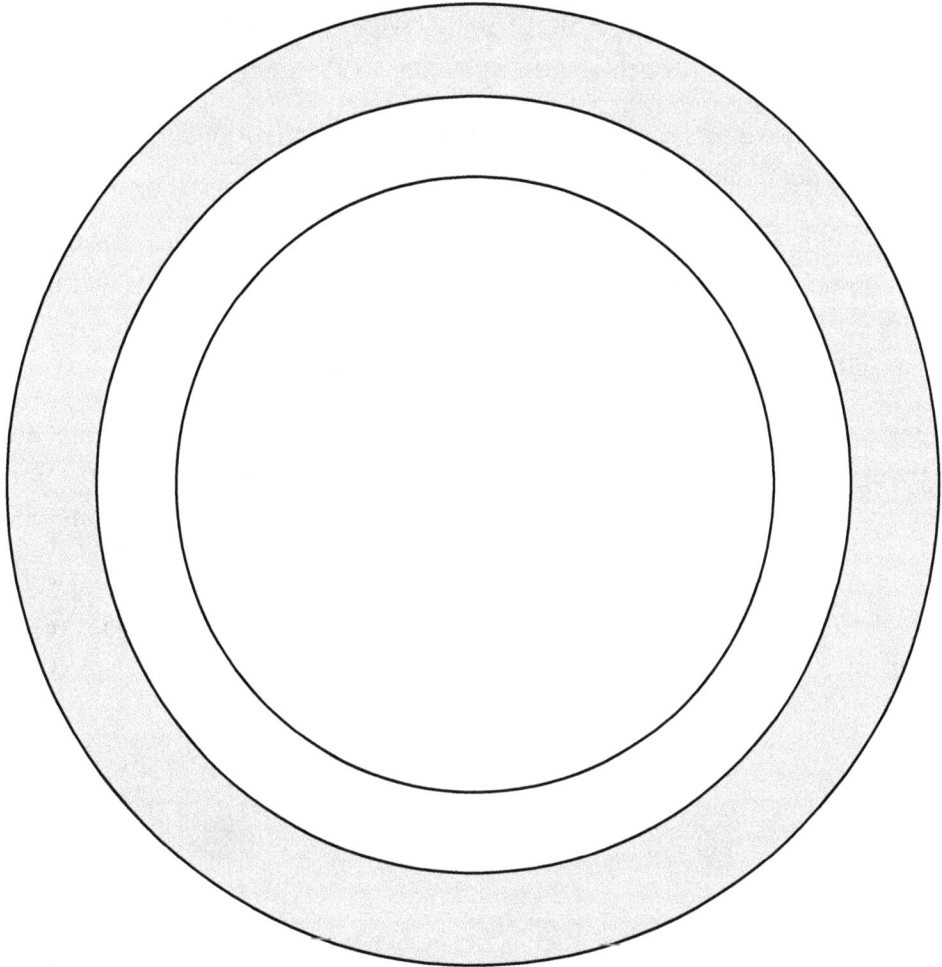

# Yup

My reaction to my encounter with Lorenzo that evening was a little more empathetic than the cop's: *Been there.*

I mean, I've only had one run-in with the police when I drank too much. And although I was a drunken nice guy too, they didn't give me a ride home.

However, I have heard lots of stories from friends about their alcohol-related missteps that resulted in police handcuffs and near arrests.

My friends and I have also made our share of messes with our significant others because we drank too much on various occasions. And then, the next day, we had to take responsibility for our actions, apologize for our insensitivities and make our relationships right again with appreciative deeds or remorseful gifts or both.

So since neither I nor any of my friends have been arrested for our excessive alcohol antics, though all of us have had plenty of arguments, hang-ups, brush-offs and silent treatments with our wives or girlfriends after we drank too much, I saw myself in Lorenzo.

My truth about the reason why Lorenzo's day turned out the way it did was: *Yup, he drank too much.*

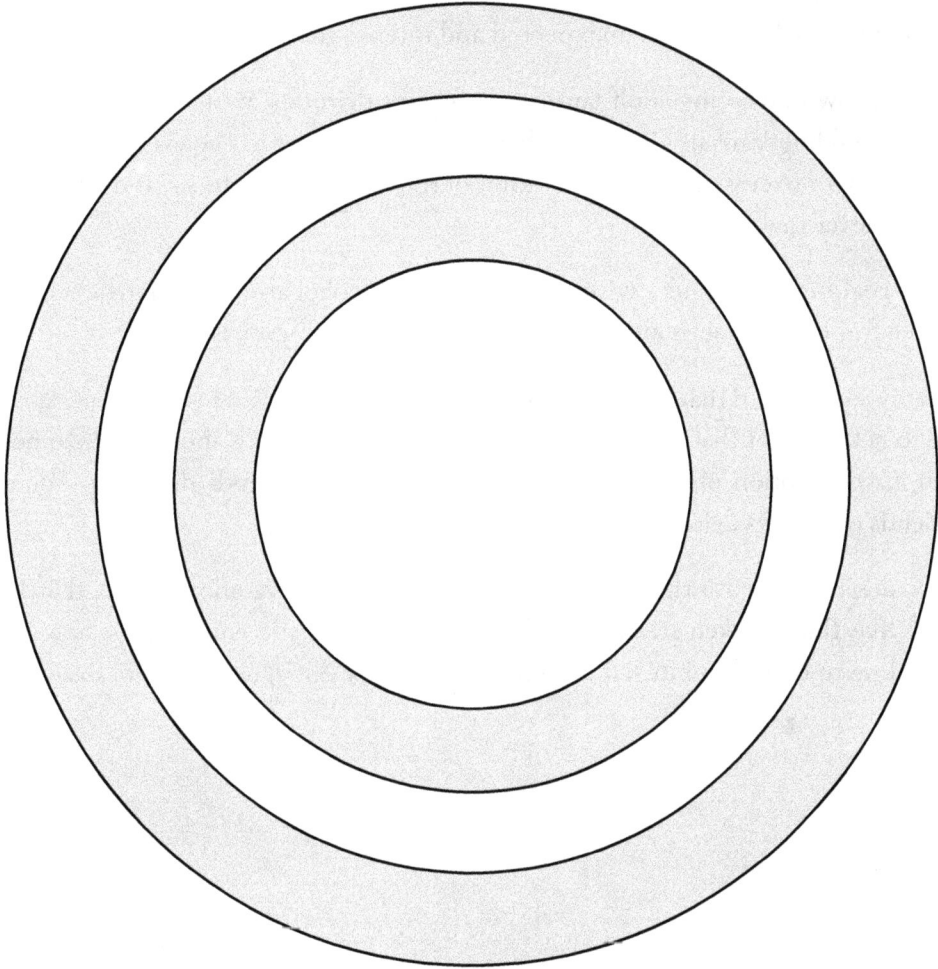

# SMH

My son's new opinion of Lorenzo because of the disturbing situation he witnessed that night: *Idiot*.

After a ton of thought about his unexpected and intense reaction, I figured it out.

My son has grown up seeing adult family and friends drinking at birthday parties and bar-beques and weddings and all kinds of gatherings. But not once has he ever seen someone he knew drinking to excess or making any kind of mess. That's not to say it didn't happen—just that he never saw it.

In fact, his real-life experiences with adults drinking alcohol around him matched the same drama-free fun he's also seen all his life in the alcohol commercials on TV.

So when my son learned that Lorenzo's drinking had caused police involvement, and caused his wife to get so upset that she didn't want to help him, his truth about Lorenzo no longer matched his perception of safe, smart and fun family and friends drinking—or even of adult friends of friends drinking.

The only alternative truth that his limited teenage perspective allowed was that Lorenzo had to be like the drunken strangers he'd begun seeing while enjoying his new hobby of surfing online to entertain himself with internet videos: *SMH, old enough to know better.*

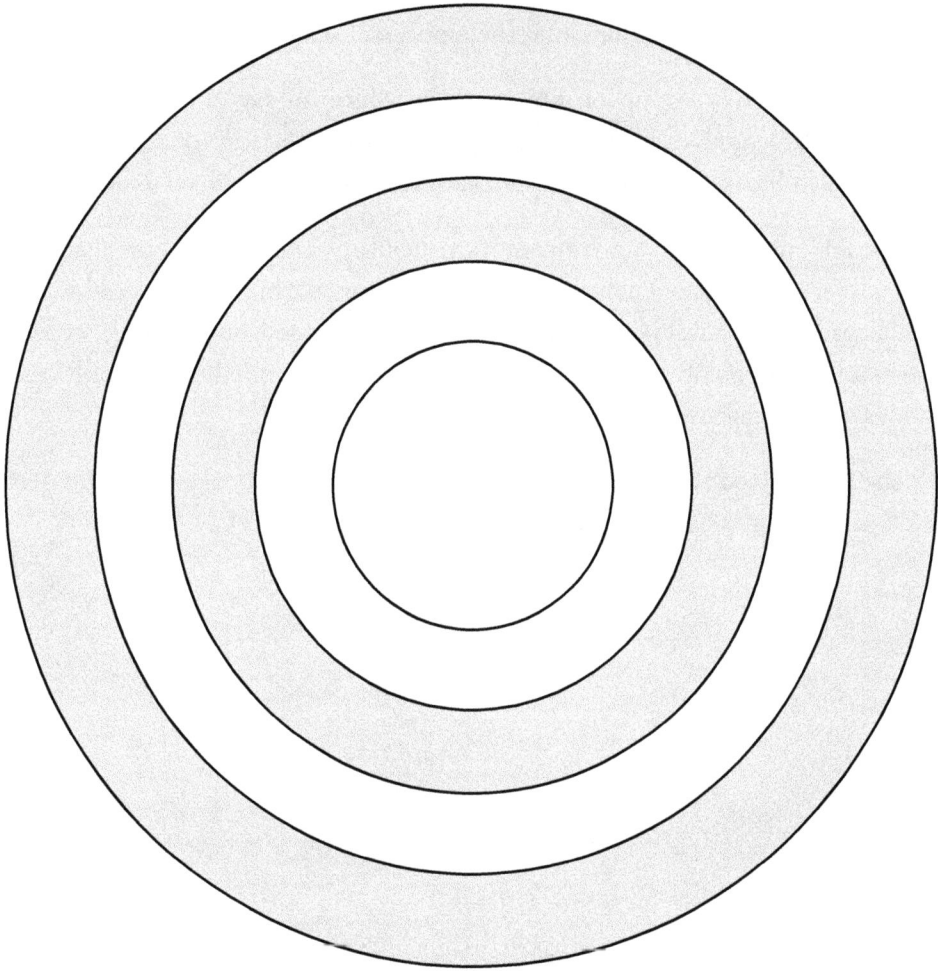

# Grrrr

My guess about Camilla's reaction was that it was similar to my son's in intensity. However, hers seemed way further along the emotional scale of disappointment: *Enough*.

For her to immediately hang up on him after hearing him say one word to her from a number she didn't recognize, it seemed likely this was not the first or second or fifth time Lorenzo had called her to help him clean up another one of his drinking messes.

She had probably already learned from every other time she helped him that despite his promises and her efforts, her husband's attempts to correct his behavior did not last. She had likely already been understanding and helpful, surprised but helpful, impatient but helpful, frustrated but helpful, angry but helpful—but each time her help only resulted in Lorenzo making another mess again anyway.

And now she had arrived at the ultimate level of disappointment: obstinate and dismissive. Camilla's truth was simple: *Grrrr, just control yourself already.*

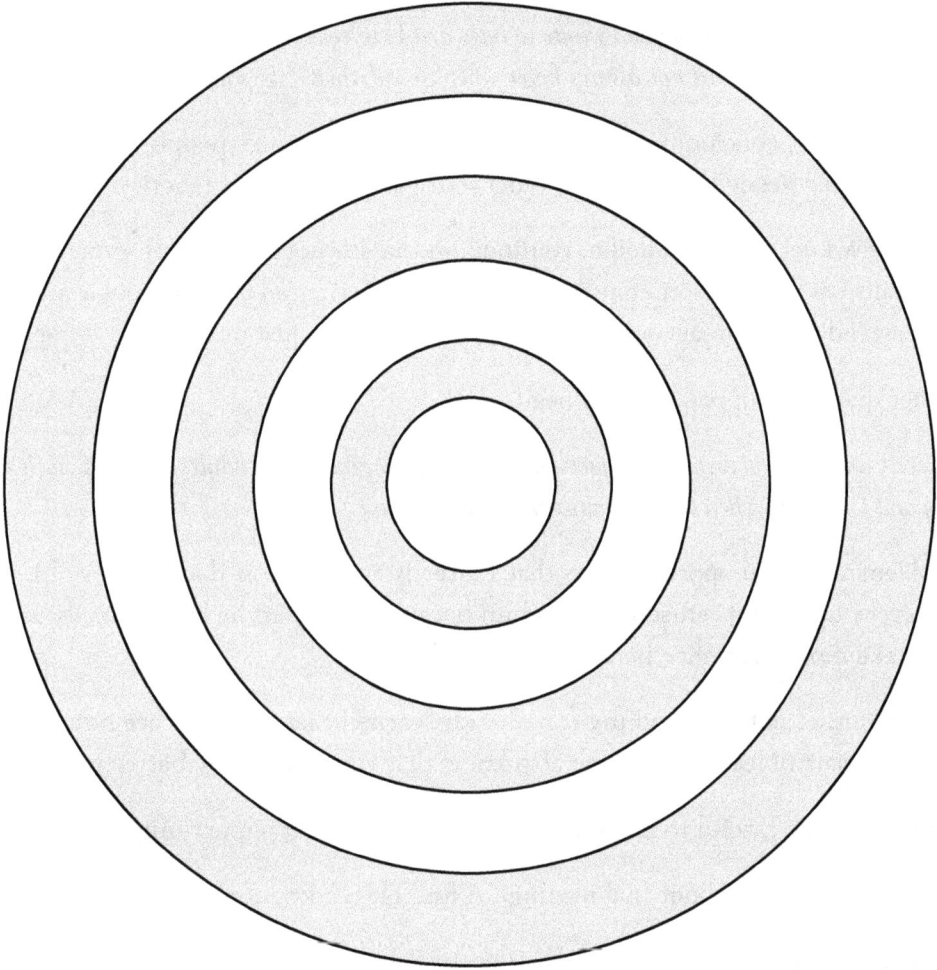

# Shrug

So as I continued to think about what all of our different interpretations meant during our evening together, a question popped into my head.

*If Lorenzo is so smart and capable and wants to have drinks to celebrate his accomplishments, like most of us also do, then why does he not always know when to say when, like some of us also do?*

And instead of just concluding like I always had that sometimes people mistakenly drank too much and just needed a little help, I focused again on my son's reaction.

I mean, I knew I definitely needed to remind him that it's not nice to call someone an idiot, nor is it healthy to dismiss someone as stupid. But I also wanted to figure out a way to make him understand that his reaction wasn't wrong, but rather, just not entirely complete.

So another question popped into my head.

*Should I tell my son that drinking is just part of being an adult, and adults just help each other by forgiving and forgetting when we make mistakes with alcohol?*

The problem with that approach was that I already told my son that I believed Lorenzo's wife was very upset and refused to help him because it seemed he had probably made that same mistake more than once before.

And in our house, not only had my son already learned that mistakes are not bad and are an important part of learning, but he also knew that when we know better we do better.

I needed to be very careful to not sidestep this huge teaching opportunity for my son.

So I continued thinking about that evening. A lot. Then a lot more after that.

Every angle. Every detail. Then, finally, it occurred to me.

There was another perspective that drove all of our reactions that evening.

The perspective no one consciously considers, but still affects all of our reactions.

The sixth perspective during our evening——the alcohol companies: *(Shrug), told ya so.*

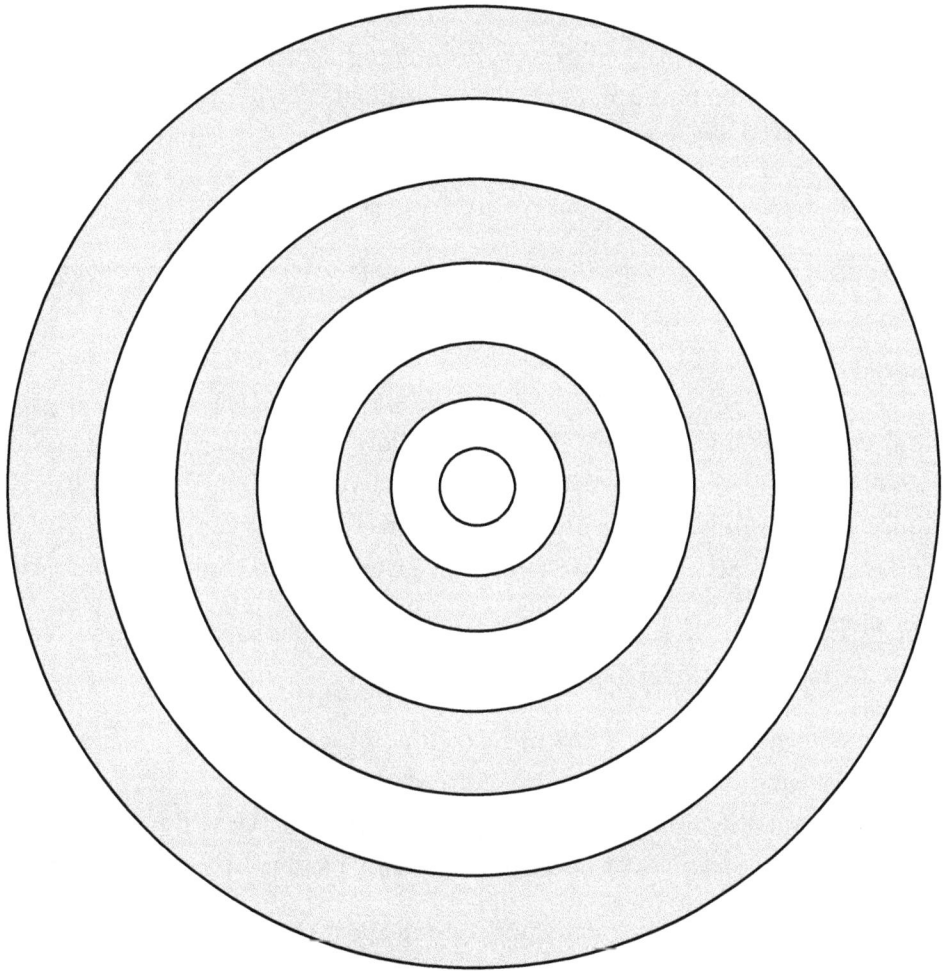

# Ah-ha!

I was jumping up and down!

I felt like I had discovered an alternate reality, like the one in *The Matrix* movie!

One story, six truths, but only one of us was drinking. I realized the five of us had each adopted a different version of the SIXTH truth—without even knowing it. So much so that we wouldn't disagree if we were to share and learn each other's version of the truth.

So what was the bottom-line truth that we all basically agreed about?

*Lorenzo didn't drink responsibly, and although he didn't mean to make a mess, he did anyway, so it's all his fault.*

Fascinating, right!?!

So why did we believe that Lorenzo just didn't follow the simple directions to drink responsibly? Why did we just dismiss what we knew about Lorenzo—that he was a smart, capable, nice guy that fully intended to drink responsibly and have a nice day that day and the other days before that? Why did we believe he just needed to choose to control himself?

Yeah, I finally figured out all the answers about why that night happened, as well as how to clarify it all for my son to understand too.

I also figured out why drinking is the most common social accessory, and why unintentional and repetitive messes caused by excessive drinking like Lorenzo's are perceived to be in-frequent even though they actually happen all the time. And I figured out why all of us can relate to the perspectives of Lorenzo and Camilla and the cop and my son and me.

Sheesh! Really good stuff to have finally understood about the world! I felt so much lighter!

But in order for me to explain it well, you're gonna have to settle in with me for a little while.

I promise it will be a fun ride kind of story, and worth your time.

But the answers are probably not what you're expecting.

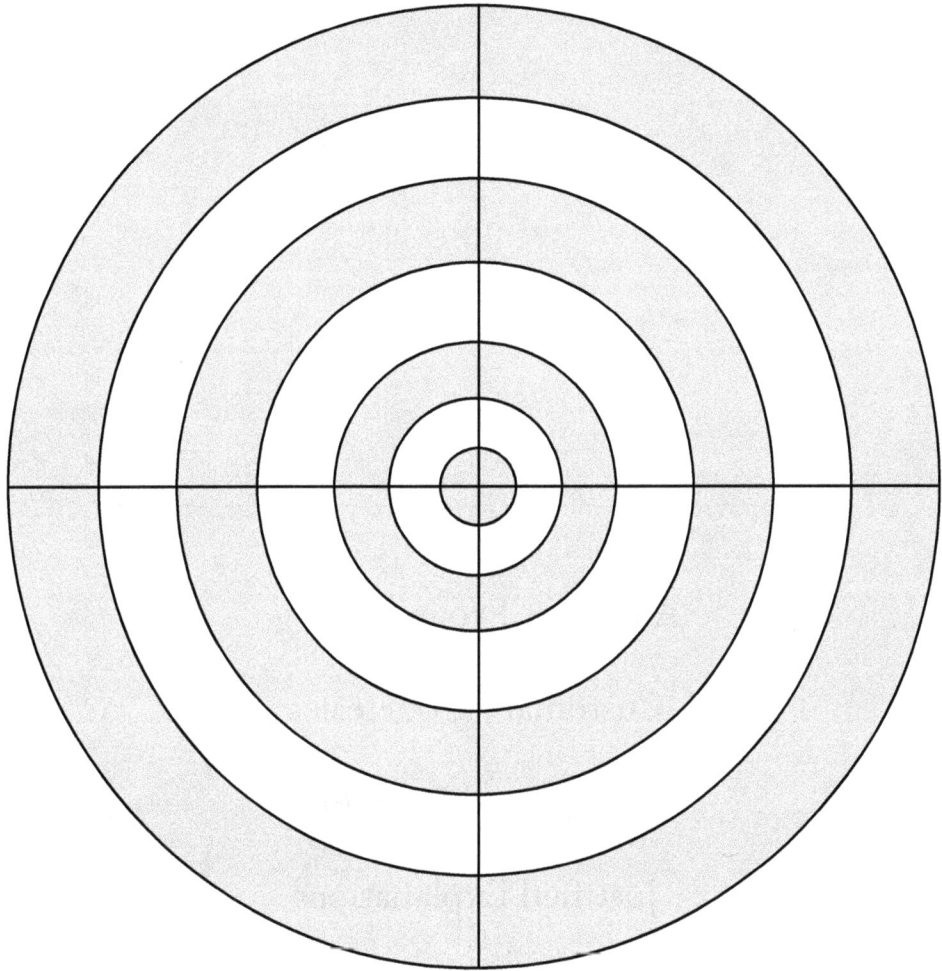

# LET'S TAKE
# A JER-NEY

Autopilot Programming

Customary Courtesies

Unexpected Reactions

Justified Explanations

Refreshed Game Plans

. . . and start all the way back
at our common childhoods

# Autopilot Programming

From the time we were kids, we've all grown up with alcohol. But I'm not talking about child-drinkers. What I'm saying is alcohol has been in our background surroundings since before we can remember and throughout our childhood memories.

Friends and family cheerfully toasted our birth; we watched from our highchairs as some of our relatives lovingly sang happy birthday to us with alcohol-looking drinks in hand, we saw Dad and the neighbors having beers while enjoying their team play on TV, we noticed Mom liked wine with her dinner conversations at large family gatherings.

And even if Mom and Dad didn't drink very often or even at all, the friends and family that Mom and Dad socialized with did, or at the very least, the celebrities they enjoyed watching on TV shows, movies and alcohol commercials did. So you get my point about alcohol being present in our lives as long as we can remember.

Most of us were also even allowed a taste of Mom's wine or a sip of Dad's beer when we asked at various times during our childhood—which only reinforced the innocence of alcohol, right? Because, since Mom and Dad drank alcohol, and they're normal and safe, then alcohol must be normal and safe too. After all, our all-knowing parents couldn't refuse us a sip of something they're drinking because it's bad—right? Or tell us that Grandpa Fred and Aunt Ginny were making the wrong choice to drink whiskey at family barbeques—right? That would have been confusing.

And when we asked for another sip because we saw Mom pour another glass of wine or Dad open another beer, the best they could do was tell us that the taste we already had was enough because alcohol is for adults.

So no wonder we all looked forward to turning 21 more than turning 18 during our most formative first two decades of life on the planet. 18 is the legal age of consent, but 21 is the legal age of consumption. At 18, the boring parts of being an adult kick in, but at 21, that's when the adult good times start to roll. Sure, we can vote and join the military at 18, and we don't have to have our Mom or Dad co-sign legal documents for us anymore. But at 21, whewwww, we can finally buy and freely join-in with alcohol drinkers everywhere it's served—which makes us feel like being an adult has always looked to us.

Hence, the foundation of our belief about drinking alcohol has been programmed into us for as long as we've been alive: it's a safe and normal way for adults to relax and have fun while socializing with each other.

Good stuff, right?! Our relationship with alcohol is innocent and simple but deeply affecting in an almost subliminal programming kind of way.

I told you this would be a fun story!

Don't worry, we're just getting started. There are all kinds of ingredients and toppings to discuss about this sundae before we even get to the cherry on top, so let's keep going.

# Customary Courtesies

After we turned 21 and could therefore drink openly and legally, the freedom we felt was like when as kids we were released from our classroom to the playground, or when we were a little older and accepted as the newest member of the most well-known but age-restricted social club.

Nothing feels better than freedom and acceptance. The feeling we got when we were first ordering, accepting, offering and holding an alcoholic beverage was as good a feeling as we were taught it would be by the zillions of fun alcohol ads we've seen and countless happy drinking experiences we watched our families have when we were growing up.

So when we arrived at social gatherings as a fresh 21-year-old, and the host asked if he could get us something to drink, we replied *YES!*—because we could!

And when we began welcoming guests as a twenty-something host of our own gatherings, not only did we offer them a drink, we also had all kinds of different alcohol to serve them. Because we learned that having alcohol to offer our guests is customary, and that having a variety of alcohol choices to serve them is courteous.

Then interestingly, as we got a little older, the freedom and acceptance club started to separate into two cliques.

Both groups continued to feel free by drinking as often and as much as they wanted. But at some point, one group began feeling more free by drinking more often and having more refills, while the other group began feeling more free by knowing that although they could drink more often and have more refills, they chose not to.

Both groups also continued to feel accepted as a normal adult with a drink in hand. But at some point, one group began impressing upon others to have a drink as their way of help-ing everyone feel accepted, while the other group felt accepted no matter how little they were drinking.

So, it's funny (or not—depending on which way you look at it) how our customary get-along skills and peer pressure strategies developed during our childhood also continue to play out as courteous social adults with alcohol.

"Dude, come have a beer with me. I know you like to run after work, but we had a tough day . . . so talking about it over a couple beers will be good for both of us."

"Ohhh Sweetie, I didn't know you wanted a girl's night because he broke up with you. After we finish our spritzers, we're switching to liquor . . . I'll have you feeling better before you know it."

"Gurrrl, what do you mean you're done drinking after one glass of wine? We're all here celebrating YOU getting into grad school . . . so I'm getting both of us another one."

Hey Mannn, I agree no drinking tonight if you think you're getting a cold, but you need to do two shots of whiskey with me right now . . . it will make both of us feel better and kill whatever bug we may have picked up."

# Unexpected Reactions

The ways people react when drinking aren't always the relaxed smiles and easy laughs we saw growing up with our parents, family friends and alcohol ads.

In addition to our newfound feelings of freedom and acceptance while socializing openly with alcohol after we turn 21, we are also surprised when we start seeing that drinking alcohol sometimes causes people to behave differently than we expect. And sometimes it doesn't have anything to do with how much or how often someone drinks.

The bottom line is that when people are drinking, no one really knows if anything out of the ordinary is gonna happen, but it might.

"Thanks for having the whole family over to your place for a such a fun birthday barbeque for Cousin Tim last weekend. The best part was when quiet Uncle Peter surprised everyone by having a couple vodkas then taking off his clothes and walking around in his boxers, undershirt and knee-high dress socks telling stories about his younger days as a hippie hair stylist. So much fun. Too bad Aunt Debbie made them both leave as soon as she saw him after she got back with the chicken wings."

"Yeah, I'm really embarrassed with myself and I'm pissed at you. Our bar crawl started out so great last night. I remember finally approaching that hot girl that I've been seeing out for weeks. Then I wake up this morning to a text from her telling me I'm blocked. So I scroll up to see a text close-up pic of my belly button that you must have sent her after I passed out. I don't even know what that means. I thought you were my friend, Man."

"Hey, it's better that you were studying for your college exams and couldn't make it to last night's family dinner. We were all celebrating Granny and Grampy's anniversary and thanking them for always being so kind and generous, then for some reason Mom ordered a martini, and the positive conversation quickly turned into everyone consoling Mom's tears about Granny and Grampy making her childhood so difficult. None of us saw that awkwardness coming."

"What do you mean you don't know why that huge MMA-looking guy bloodied your nose with his elbow in the stadium men's room?"

# Justified Explanations

When the unexpected and unintended drinking experiences do happen, we simply revert back to what we learned as kids. We explain it away as a non-event. Why? Because that's what we heard our parents do. And because any drinking experience that doesn't match the good times that the alcohol company ads show us must be an anomaly attributable to something or someone other than their product.

Life is a matter of perspective. Attitude is everything. Everybody deserves a second chance. Right? Right. So we justified or forgot about our sideways alcohol experiences, and then got back to making the good times roll again.

"Are you saying that Uncle Peter has been taking off his pants and telling his hippie stories at our family gatherings longer than I've been alive?! Wow. You guys always told me when I noticed they were suddenly gone from dinner with everyone was because Uncle Peter got hot and Aunt Debbie had to take him home to cool down. I guess that isn't a lie. It's just that no one wanted to explain his harmless drunken fun to the kids. Hm . . . Okay."

"Ohhhh, I'm the one that sent that girl I just met the pic of my belly button last night?! Before I threw up? Thanks for not letting me puke in my bed. And I'm glad to know that hot girl doesn't have a sense of humor before I spent any money on her. Phew, it was a good night after all."

" What?! I didn't know Mom got drunk that night to finally confront Granny and Grampy for drinking so much and ruining her childhood. I had no idea, but I hear you, Dad. There's no reason to talk about that trauma anymore. What's passed is in the past, and we're just gonna focus on being happy going forward—got it. "

"You're right—the MMA-looking guy definitely didn't need to elbow your face. So you peed on his shoe at the urinal next to yours. It was an honest mistake—his flame socks looked real and you were just trying to help. The good news is your bloody nose isn't broken. Come on, just hold that paper towel on your nose and let's get back to our seats."

# Refreshed Game Plans

The good-time-sweet-spot of relaxation and fun that alcohol promises is real. But it's not guaranteed. So we practice. And we learn from our mistakes, and the mistakes made by those around us. And we quickly learn it's up to us to figure out the proper combination of alcohol and circumstances needed to create the best chance of hitting our target drinking experience.

The good news is, that after a few hits and misses, we begin to see the pattern that leads all of our drinking stories to consistently fall into one of four easy-to-identify categories: fuzzy, good, bad, and ugly. And, from there, we can adjust our game plan to set ourselves up for success next time.

If our memories are fuzzy, we help each other make sense and feel better about the parts we don't remember so well.

If our memories are good, we pat ourselves on the back.

If our memories are bad, we downplay them.

If our memories are ugly, we resolve them with blame.

It might seem like a lot of effort to get good at drinking, but it doesn't feel like work as soon as we learn how to do it more often than not. AND it feels good to be good at something that everybody likes to do too.

It makes perfect sense that we keep coming back to drink and try to recreate the good times.

"YEAH BABY,
Sunday Booze Brunches
are my new way to relax AND
recharge! Drink, eat and socialize
like royalty all afternoon, then go home
and sleep off all the pollution for twelve
hours so I can start work like a champ
again Monday morning. My new
Sunday plan is definitely
a MUST DO!"

"I don't
remember getting
home either, Sweetie. All
good though, because I already
heard from Rich this morning.
He said he was buying us shots all
night and didn't see us do anything
embarrassing—soooo let's only
let Rich buy us beer when we
meet up there AGAIN
TONIGHT!"

"If my wife
joined me at my office
holiday party Friday night like
I wanted, she wouldn't have let me
do tequila shots with the fellas, or let
me pull my pants down and moon my
Boss from across the room—and today
I wouldn't be fired looking for a job.
Still not sure if my busy wife or
my uptight Boss is to blame
for this mess."

"No, I'm not dating
him anymore. Yes, he was
very handsome and really smart
and always trying to make me laugh
and taking me to super-nice places,
but I need to be with someone who
wants to drink and let loose with
me. I'll be fine though . . . no
biggie . . . NEXT!"

# IT'S ALL GOOD

A look for every like

A tribe for every vibe

A flavor for every taste

A place for every preference

Appropriate for every occasion

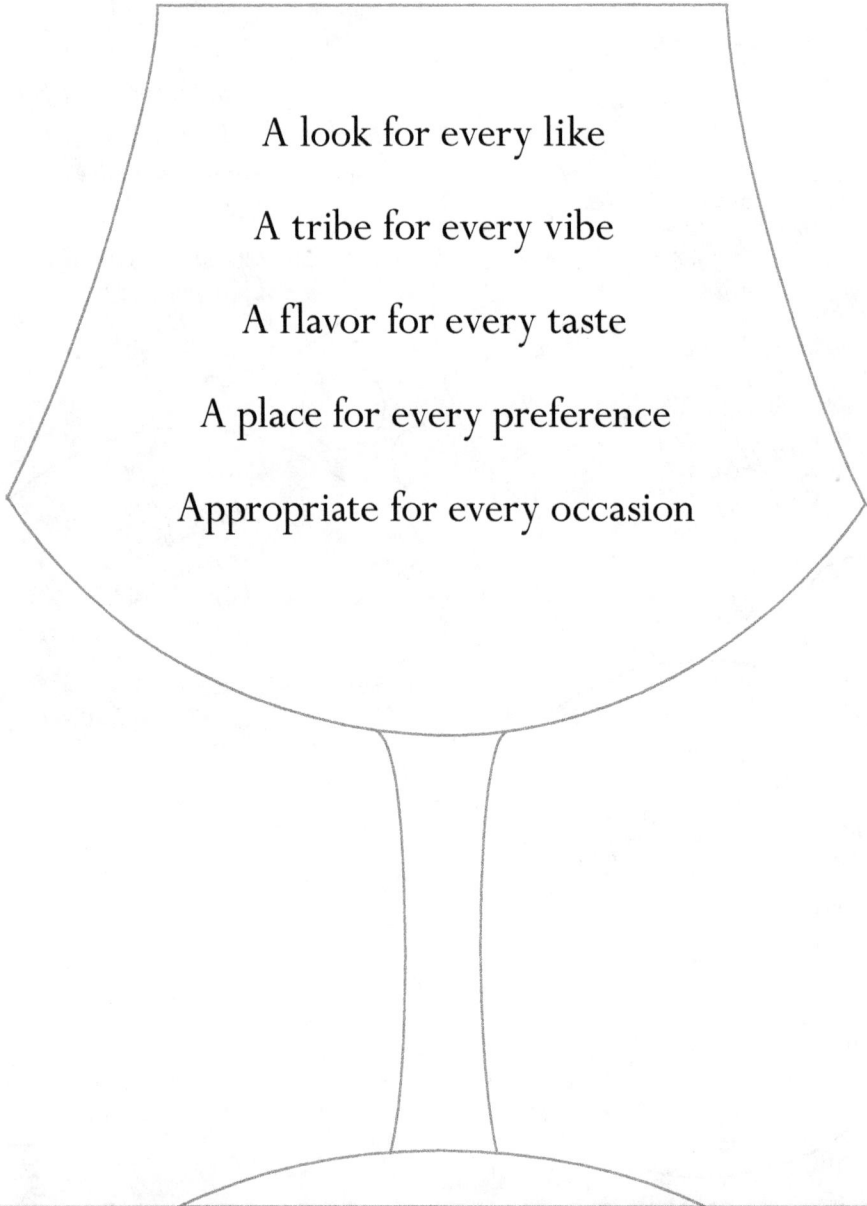

. . . so have another one!

# A Look For Every Like

The way alcohol looks when we see someone drinking is a big reason for our common attraction to drink too.

The cleverly-shaped cups and glasses in which alcohol is served draws our interest based on our mood at any particular time. Whether it's in a simple mug, sturdy stein, sophisticated chalice, fancy flute, strong shot glass, masculine martini glass or a casual plastic cup—the type of alcohol is usually a match to the unique-looking container it's served in, so it's very likely we'll also enjoy whatever we see someone else drinking.

The eye-catching textures that can be created with alcohol are often a match to the feeling we have or want. On a hot and tiring day, the sight of alcohol served as a frozen slushy looks pretty refreshing—like what you'd drink while cooling off sitting in a floating pool chair. After a heavy-stress-filled day, seeing alcohol slowly swirling around cubed ice looks kinda relaxing—like the calm view from the back porch after a storm. And on cold days, either due to winter weather or mean people, the appearance of liquor served straight-up at room temperature looks warm and soothing—just like a reassuring hug from Mom.

The exotic-looking colors of certain alcohol drink presentations make us think of sweeter times, which can be especially appealing when we're in the middle of a not-so-sweet life experience. The only thing better than seeing someone with a blue, yellow, red, or green drink is holding our own colorful alcohol refreshment as we join in with the crowd, sip with satisfaction, and beam with enjoyment too.

The fun-looking alcohol drink accessories commonly known as garnishes are not just decoration, they're also a message about the person holding it. A simple fruit wedge at the top of a beer bottle or glass makes the boring beer and ordinary drinker look more trendy and hip. Celery flowers swaying in the breeze above the rim of a tall mixer glass makes the drinker and the liquor look like they're having a wellness experience. Miniature swords tethering tiny veggie and meat pieces floating in straight liquor announces drinking heavily but responsibly, because they're also snacking.

"This ice cream birthday party is awesome for the kids, but not so much for the adults. So let's sneak a little whiskey into our root beer floats, then the adults can all scream for ice cream too!"

"Whoa! Check out that group of girls drinking from the Party Pail! Even though they look like dancing livestock around a trough, they're kinda cute, so let's get one for the table next to theirs and see if we can party with them!"

"Honey, please order each of us one of those orange shots that the bartender lights on fire, and let's get this anniversary cruise turnt-up!"

"Checkout how Dan from Accounting always has a tiny umbrella in his drink! Mannn, that guy really knows how to shift gears and relax! I'll have what he's having—WITH an umbrella, please!"

# A Tribe For Every Vibe

Since drinking is usually enjoyed as a social activity, we tend to have the best drinking experiences when everyone in our group finds each other attractive, agreeable and relatable.

The way a group is dressed is an easy indicator that we'll likely enjoy our time drinking together. Professional shirts and shiny shoes people usually find their way to a celebratory drink together—no matter what kind of work was accomplished that day. Floral shirts and slip-on sandals people usually gravitate to have a relaxing drink together—even when they're not on vacation. Player jerseys and sports logo people usually discover each other across a crowded room to toast wins or losses—especially when the crowd is for the opposing team. Trendy accessories and cool clothing people usually find their way to raise their glasses to each other's impressiveness—because admiration and alcohol mix well together.

And after we find an attractive-looking group to drink with, the next thing we do is listen and decide whether we can have a pleasant conversation together. Although you might think it's important to stick to light topics like current weather and favorite colors to have a good time drinking, it's actually the opposite that's true. As soon as we test each other's opinions about business, movies, music or sports, we can then move on to the heavier topics for a way more fun drinking experience. And it doesn't matter how much anyone in the group knows about the topic or each other. The most important ingredient for a pleasant conversation over drinks is that everyone agrees with each other.

The last important thing that brings the whole good time drinking tribe together again and again is for everyone to have the same drinking style. A group of suits drinking to their common view about office restrooms rules is a nice time, but the real civil rights bonding starts when everyone agrees to pick up the pace and switch to shots. The large after-work crowd that regularly gathers for happy hour and shop talk is an effective team building experience, but the real hard core team builders are the few that drink and shop talk long after the happy hour crowd has gone home. The line of campers in front of a micro-brewery waiting overnight to buy the newest release of limited production beer are definitely committed beer enthusiasts, but only the true brew connoisseurs will reconnect with each other later to savor the pop of robust flavors, smell the bouquet of subtle aromas, and admire the beauty of rich colors that can only be discussed properly among alcohol experts.

"That's a fabulous purse. I have one in black. Worth every dollar to not look like another basic Bea, right?! Mind if I join you? I'm having another white wine spritzer too!"

"Yeah, order me in for the next round. We'll be right back. Goin' out to the parking lot for a minute. All this self-defense talk has me fired up! Lenny's gonna show me what he carries in his trunk!"

"Partying with thousands of clothing optional people at Fantasy Fest is a blast! And it's the only time of year we get to drink like RockStars for four days straight away from our kids! My wife's greatest joy is walking around in public wearing only paint— with me by her side wearing only a sock!"

# A Flavor For Every Taste

Taste is a completely personal experience, and therefore pretty much pointless to argue about. The good news is there are so many alcohol drinks to choose from, it's also pointless to argue why you're not drinking.

The alcohol companies have done an excellent job of adding tons of different flavors to their standard beers, wines and liquors. From the increasing selection of fruity beers, tangy wines and candy liquors to the expanding variety of hard ciders, stiff sodas and spiked lemonades, the alcohol companies have made it very easy for us to choose alcohol no matter what our taste preference.

When there isn't a specific flavor made by the alcohol companies to satisfy our unique alcohol craving, well then we just add a splash of soda, a twist of fruit—or even a mix of juice, water or milk to get the drink to taste the way we want. And of course, since bartenders and mixologists are all professionally trained to know how to satisfy even the most obscure requests, all we have to do is describe the taste of the drink we want, and then watch as they masterfully pull all the ingredients together to pour us our glass of magic.

For those of us who are very particular about how the age and origin of alcohol effects the taste of our drinks, the alcohol manufacturers include this info on their labels to help us know exactly what to order. Our beer cans and bottles have *Born on* dates to let us know how freshly made they are. The year on our whiskey and wine bottles tells us how perfectly aged they are. And because all alcohol types are made and distributed all over the world, the labels also make it easy for those of us who think it's important to choose foreign or domestic.

And for the longest time, the only alcohol we could have while also trying to lose weight was light beer. So since not everybody likes beer, but more and more people are watching their weight, the alcohol companies were kind enough to start manufacturing a myriad of diet-friendly alcohol choices. And now we can choose from all kinds of flavors of low-carb beers, skinny liquors, booze waters and fit wines—guilt-free!

"I know you told me to get you a sweet-flavor beer, but they have twenty-two flavors on tap and sixteen different bottled flavors at this heavenly place. So you're gonna have to look at the menu and help me to help you, Fella!"

"Yeah, it looks cool. Got a spicy kick to it too. I didn't know what I wanted to drink, so I just grabbed a phrase from Urban Dictionary and asked the bartender to make it as if it was a real top-shelf tequila drink. And he did! It's called a Mexican Starfish!"

"Yes, I'll be home soon, Honey. Sheila and I just stopped at the bar next to our spin class for a couple skinny Cosmo's and girl talk to celebrate our new workout lifestyle before we head home for some kale and walnuts."

"Raw American oysters and real Russian vodka . . . it's the best way to celebrate foreign policy on the 4th of July—in my mouth!"

# A Place For Every Preference

No matter how we feel or wanna feel, when we wanna go out and have a drink over it, there are usually plenty of places nearby to choose from that match our preference.

High energy drinking places tend to center around activities that don't require too much concentration or coordination—so we can continue doing them while drinking and talking with our friends.

Sports Bars are fun because they have pool tables and dart boards and other games that we can keep playing pretty well while drinking and having fun arguments about whatever sports are on the giant screens throughout these places.

Nightclubs are the place to go when we want to close-talk in the dark over the loud music while drinking and dancing among crowds of strangers, pulsing lights and fantasy fog. Strip Clubs are the perfect place for times when we have money to spend on a group dating experience in a nightclub setting, but don't wanna bother with small talk or foreplay to get multiple dates to dance naked for us. Gambling places and alcohol go really well together, because drinking makes winning feel even more exciting and makes losing feel not so bad.

Calm energy drinking places offer an atmosphere that's more conducive to conversation and contemplation, so we can catch up with friends, vent about losses, brag about successes, and decide next steps.

Simple places with names like *Bar* are good spots to go when we wanna be with other people but left alone to enjoy some drinks in peace. Fancy places with lots of lighting and mirrors are the right choice when we wanna see and be seen drinking among the beautiful people and décor. Smoking places are hard to find but so satisfying when we just want to relax with a drink and a smoke inside like the old days. Neighborhood places are comforting because everybody knows our name and we can always find somebody to talk to.

Family-friendly drinking places are not just limited to restaurants and resorts anymore. When we wanna go out drinkin AND enjoy some family fun, there are plenty of places to eat, drink and be merry—WITH the kids along.

Movie theaters are popping up all over where we can have a full food and bar menu delivered right to our reclining seats, and then either enjoy the movie with the kids or nod off without them noticing. Bowling alleys are now being built with nightclub music and lighting for the lanes, sports bar screens and games areas for all interests, and wandering servers delivering cocktails and mocktails for all ages. The sip and paint places are becoming very popular because they provide an excellent cultural experience for our kids to learn about art, while the Moms and Dads learn about wine.

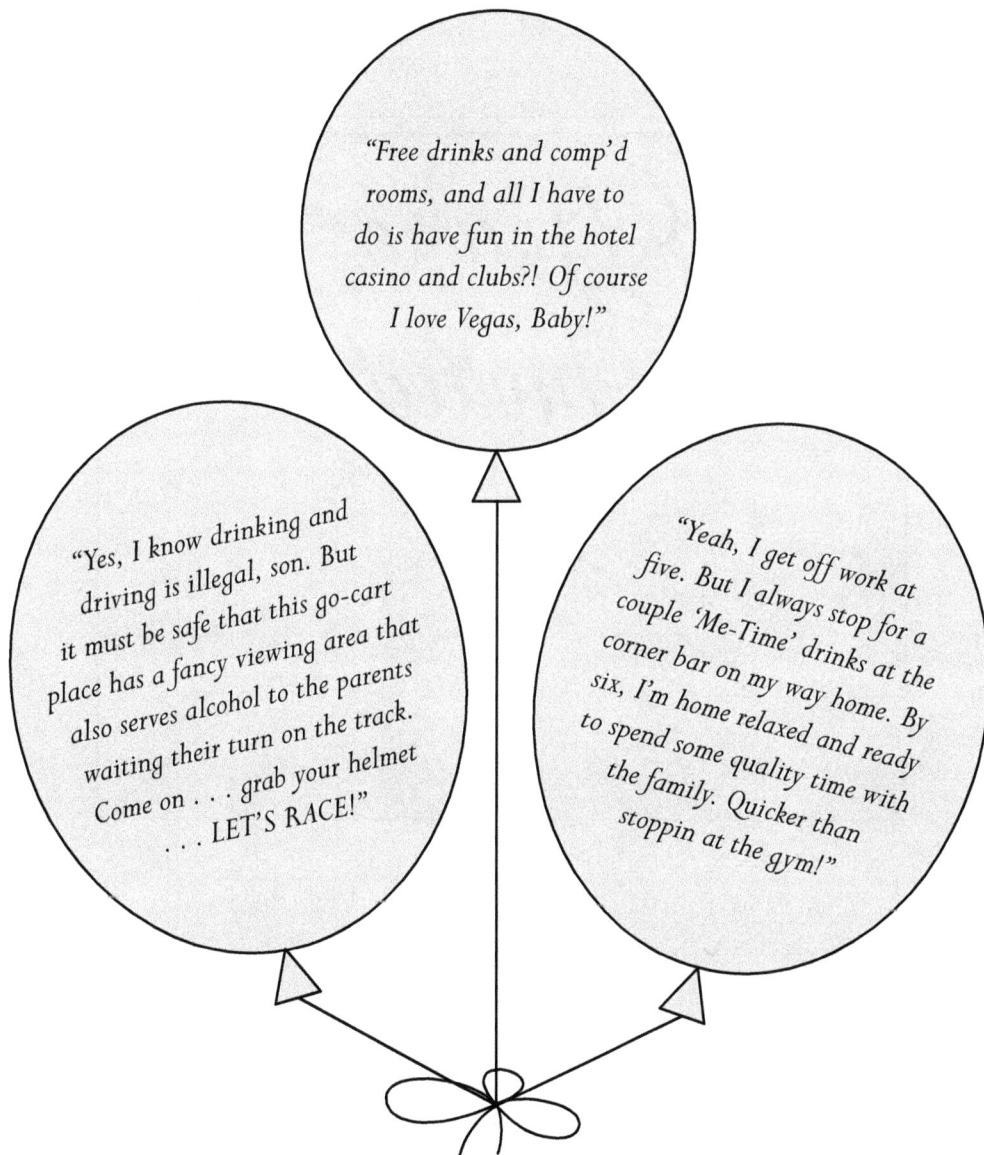

*"Free drinks and comp'd rooms, and all I have to do is have fun in the hotel casino and clubs?! Of course I love Vegas, Baby!"*

*"Yes, I know drinking and driving is illegal, son. But it must be safe that this go-cart place has a fancy viewing area that also serves alcohol to the parents waiting their turn on the track. Come on . . . grab your helmet . . . LET'S RACE!"*

*"Yeah, I get off work at five. But I always stop for a couple 'Me-Time' drinks at the corner bar on my way home. By six, I'm home relaxed and ready to spend some quality time with the family. Quicker than stoppin at the gym!"*

# Appropriate For Every Occasion

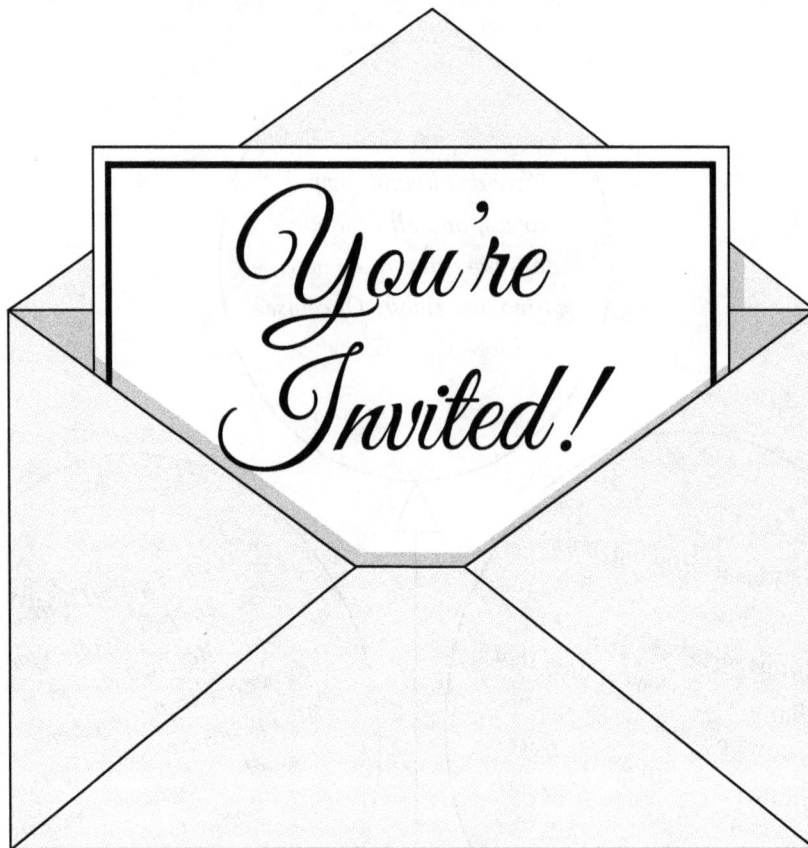

*You're Invited!*

| | |
|---|---:|
| Holiday | Girls' Night |
| Birthday | Guys' Trip |
| Anniversary | Started Dating |
| Wedding | Stopped Dating |
| Funeral | Fell in Love |
| Just Hired | Fell Out of Love |
| Just Fired | Just Immigrated |
| Just Retired | Just Deported |
| Just Married | Accepted to College |
| Just Separated | Graduated from College |
| Just Divorced | Kicked Out of College |
| Job Promotion | Passed the Test |
| Job Demotion | Failed the Test |
| Pay Raise | Found Guilty |
| Pay Cut | Found Innocent |
| Convicted | Thank God it's Friday |
| Paroled | Monday Sucks |
| Engaged | Sunny Day |
| Abandoned | Rainy Day |
| Won the Game | Boozy Brunch |
| Lost the Game | Liquid Lunch |

*Alcohol . . . it's always a good time for a drink.*

# UNTIL IT'S NOT

Offensive Words

Embarrassing Actions

Uncontrollable Ailments

Unforeseen Consequences

. . . so no more for you!

# Offensive Words

The first sign that we're beginning to have too much to drink is the way we start talking—we just don't realize we sound different.

After having a certain amount of drinks, some of us get a little hearing impaired. And this causes our speech to become progressively louder—even though the room hasn't gotten any noisier or the person we're talking with hasn't moved any further away. Alcohol impaired hearing also causes our story punctuations and reactions to start bursting out of us—as if everything we say and hear is a howling punchline.

Alcohol can also start to have a clouding affect on our choice of stories and reactions too. It's not much fun to meet up for drinks after work and have to listen to our friend complaining about their dead-end job situation and crying about their stalled relationship situation. Or when that friend finally asks about us and hears that we're doing fine, and then reacts with agitation instead of congratulation.

When some of us continue to mix more alcohol with our otherwise normal ability to remain calm and patient, our string of passive reactions can suddenly turn into aggressive and dismissive ultimatums.

Declining sensitivity toward the people nearby is another way we can tell that someone is beginning to have a few too many drinks. This can sometimes lead to startlingly disrespectful comments, and even vulgar remarks.

"Dude, switch barstools with me before Kyle gets back from the men's room. I just can't handle sitting next to him anymore. It's like listening to a jet engine blowing on and off in my face!"

"Calm down because everyone's looking over here?! You invited ME to catchup over drinks! But all YOU wanna do is talk about how great everything is going for YOU!"

"Yeah, I heard you tell him I got fat! Remember to also tell him you don't make anywhere near the money you did when I agreed to marry you! Just make me another martini and shut up, Jackass! Or else I'll start smoking again!"

I like how your sweater fits. Never met you before, but if my granddaughter brings you to another of these family get-togethers, I just want you to know you're okay with me.

# Embarrassing Actions

After a few more drinks, in addition to sounding different, some of us begin behaving differently too, which we may not realize even when we become embarrassing to ourselves and others.

The relaxing effect that alcohol has on our heavy thoughts can also have a numbing effect on our physical awareness. His open zipper, her gaping blouse, his drooping drawers, and her skirt tucked into her thong are not always the result of too much alcohol, but they're all way more likely with a few too many drinks in us.

As the drinks continue to flow, those of us who have a normally welcoming-friendly nature can sometimes start to get a little too touchy-friendly with the people nearby. High-fiving the strangers that aren't even watching the big screen, or kissing the hand of the waitress bringing our cocktails may seem to like normal friendliness, but can be perceived as creepy by those around us that are not also on their third round.

And as alcohol's effects continue to move us along from relaxed to overly-friendly, the next feel-good we experience is usually high-energy-confidence. Again, this is awesome for us and everyone around us at the right time and place, but not so much when Dads start jumping off the roof into the pool at their nine-year-old's birthday party, or when co-workers decide to play Beer Pong in the main conference room following the annual company meeting.

Then, inevitably, the combination of alcohol and high energy antics makes us so tired that we can only manage low-effort solutions to any problems that arise. Hungry? Any fast food will do. Tired of holding your phone? Into your bra it goes. Sore feet on the dance floor? Just kick off your heels. Long line to the Ladies Restroom? Use the Men's Restroom. No restroom in sight? Gotta pee in public.

"Whoa! Check it out! Lisa's left boob has slipped completely out of her bikini! No wonder all the guys keep bringing her more drinks! We should go over and help. But first, let me get a selfie with her!"

"Okay honey, Robert just switched from beer to whiskey, so that's our cue to get going. He's a ton of fun to party with until he starts groping and petting the wrong guy's wife or girlfriend. I'd rather avoid another bar brawl when Robert tries to argue he's just being friendly."

"On the left side of the room, we have Pauly, who is attempting his second jump over an office chair without spilling his beer. On the right side of the room, we have Ann, who is holding two beers so Staci can use both her hands to properly flash everyone the results of her breast enhancement surgery. In the doorway, we have our Boss, who is clearly not amused. It's like watching a slow-motion train wreck . . . not gonna end well, but I can't look away!"

"Hey Dad! We need you outside! A few minutes ago, Uncle Rick walked into the pool completely clothed, and is now laying on a pool float peeing straight up like a fountain in front of the whole family. I guess all the drinks and emotion in this summer heat made him so hot and exhausted that he forgot he's at Grandma Jean's funeral."

# Uncontrollable Ailments

For whatever reason, sometimes our friends don't tell us to slow or stop drinking earlier when begin talking and behaving differently. Eventually, the uncontrollable effects of having even more alcohol then become ugly-obvious.

At this point, our loud stories, crying complaints and distasteful remarks begin to sound increasingly slurred as they come out of our mouths. And even though we can't hear ourselves whine and garble our words, our friends with less alcohol in them can tell that things just went from bad to worse.

The physical inabilities that usually accompany our alcohol-slurred speech are commonly known as sway-standing and wobble-walking. This is the time when keeping our balance is very important, because once we lose our center, we're likely goin down.

And, on the rare occasions that we can sway over and fall into a seat without damaging anything, the alcohol-induced spin vision and vomiting may still be on its way.

There are also other rare occasions when we've had way too much to drink and went straight from slurring to sleeping. Which may seem like good news for us, because we didn't make any messes. But it may be worse news for our friends, if we fell asleep in a not-so-good place.

"I'm fiiiiiine . . . I have-ENT had too much TO-DRINK! Leee-meee ALONE! NO! SAID-I'M-FINE!"

"I told you to keep Cousin Randy away from the wedding cake! He's been wobbling around drinking straight from that champagne bottle since we did the big toast! I knew he would fall eventually! How are the bride and groom supposed to cut the cake now that it's all over Randy on the floor?!"

"Oh good, Irvine made it back to the hotel lobby. Oh man . . . he just put his drink down and raised his hands as if to balance himself while he's sitting! He's definitely got the spins. Whoops! He just threw up on himself."

"Aw geez, I found Kerry. I can see her through the crack in the stall. Sitting on the toilet. Pants down. Drink in hand resting on her knee. Passed out. One of us is going to have to crawl under the stall on this gross restroom floor and unlock the door so we can pull up her jeans and carry her out."

# Unforeseen Consequences

The morning that follows our outta control drinking experience is best summarized in one word: consequences. Because unfortunately, the more we drank the day before to relax our thoughts or turn up the party, the greater the likelihood that our consequences are not limited to waking up on our couch fully dressed with a terrible headache.

Sometimes we wake up not knowing where we are. Opening our eyes to see that we slept naked hugging a toilet can be confusing until we see our drink on the vanity next to the picture of our mother and realize we're home in our own bathroom. But the relief of knowing we're home is short-lived when we walk into our bedroom in shock to see a naked man and woman we don't recognize smiling from our bed.

Other mornings, after we regain our energy to move around a little bit, we discover the damage caused by one or more too-much-fun-drinks. Then we have to figure out how to make everything right again.

Sometimes it's not possible to make it right, and we just have to live with the consequences that our excessive drinking created. Like waking up to see that we placed 67 unanswered calls to our Ex. Or checking social media to see we were tagged in pics someone posted of our bar fight and sleeping in our own vomit in the hotel lobby.

"Hi Lisa. I'm Dan. This is Rose. Oh . . . your bikini is over there. Super fun rave last night, huh? Thanks for inviting us back to your place. Got any cereal? You really know how to make a guy and girl hungry!"

"You're sorry?! You'll fix it?! Shut up! Your daughter's ninth birthday party not enough fun for you, huh?! You and your buddies just had to keep jumping off the roof into the pool, right?! Don't talk to me. Just call and get the hole in our roof fixed. And clean all your blood off the patio chair you passed out in! Then order me this diamond bracelet online! And go apologize to your daughter!"

"Yes, Mom, I'm okay. Yes, I saw the pictures online. No, I'm not in jail. Yes, I'll post something now that lets all of our family and friends know too. Just gotta make this important apology call first."

# JUST DRINK
# RESPONSIBLY

Advertised Almost Everywhere We Look

Available For Sale Almost Everywhere We Go

The Most Effective Product Packaging On The Planet

The Most Brilliant Product Tagline Of All Time

*. . . but it's not as easy as they say*

# Advertised Almost Everywhere We Look

Watching the big game in the comfort of our own living room, we see the TV ads letting us know that even though we're at home, we can still feel connected to the awesome game experience because we're drinking the same beer as all the other super fans at our favorite team's stadium.

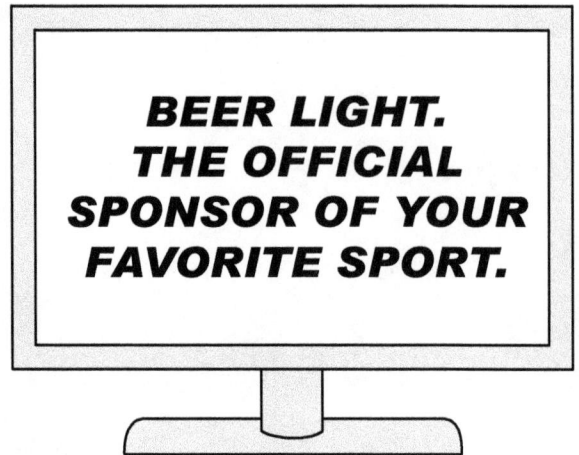

**BEER LIGHT. THE OFFICIAL SPONSOR OF YOUR FAVORITE SPORT.**

Trying to be patient while sitting in traffic, we see the giant billboard ads with our favorite celebrities encouraging us to buy a bottle of congratulations on our way home and imagine toasting with them to our worthwhile commutes to and from our important jobs.

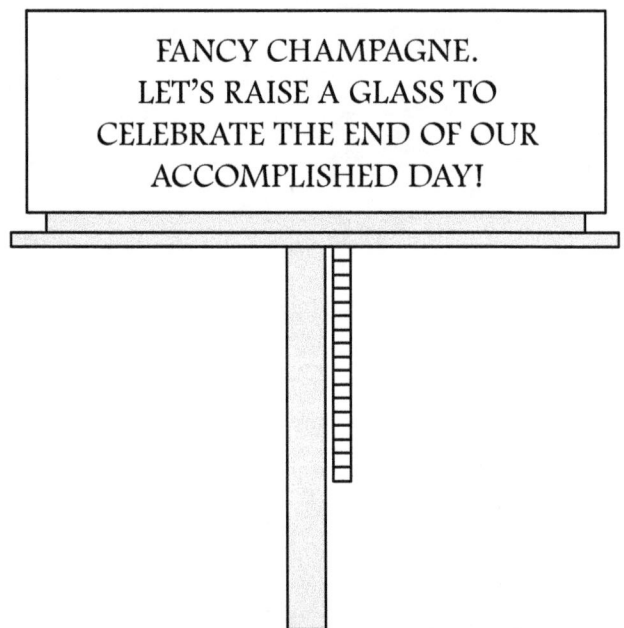

FANCY CHAMPAGNE. LET'S RAISE A GLASS TO CELEBRATE THE END OF OUR ACCOMPLISHED DAY!

Thumbing through magazines to distract our thoughts from the sounds and smells before our dental procedure, we see the beautiful beach people with perfect smiles in the glossy alcohol ads reminding us that we can stop on our way home and buy a six-pack of vacation smiles too.

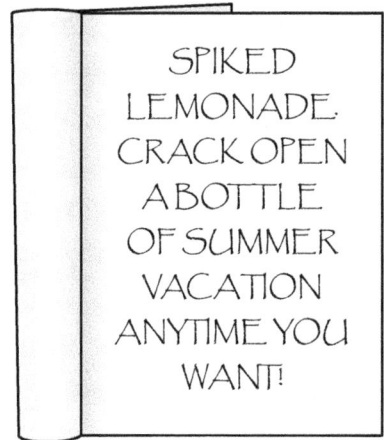

SPIKED LEMONADE. CRACK OPEN A BOTTLE OF SUMMER VACATION ANYTIME YOU WANT!

Surfing around the internet on a lazy weekend afternoon, we see the banner ads showing us how much more relaxing our day would be if we clicked to have a nice bottle of wine delivered and relocated outside with our laptop and glass of vine-ripened joy.

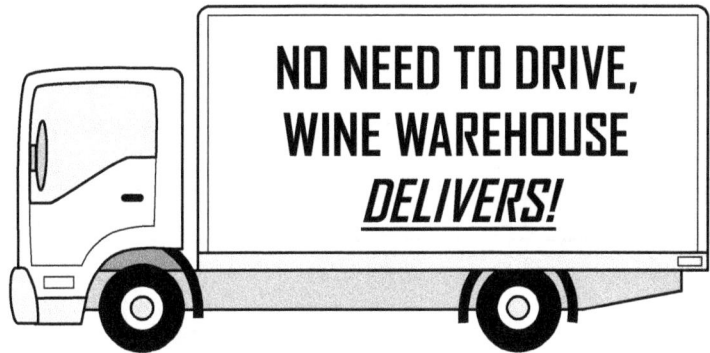

NO NEED TO DRIVE, WINE WAREHOUSE *DELIVERS!*

Checking the mail when we get home, we see the alcohol post card announcing that our local grocer has just opened an adjacent liquor store with an invitation to stop by.

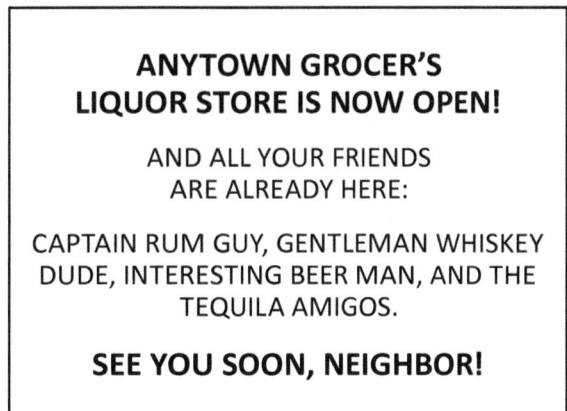

**ANYTOWN GROCER'S LIQUOR STORE IS NOW OPEN!**

AND ALL YOUR FRIENDS ARE ALREADY HERE:

CAPTAIN RUM GUY, GENTLEMAN WHISKEY DUDE, INTERESTING BEER MAN, AND THE TEQUILA AMIGOS.

**SEE YOU SOON, NEIGHBOR!**

# Available For Sale Almost Everywhere We Go

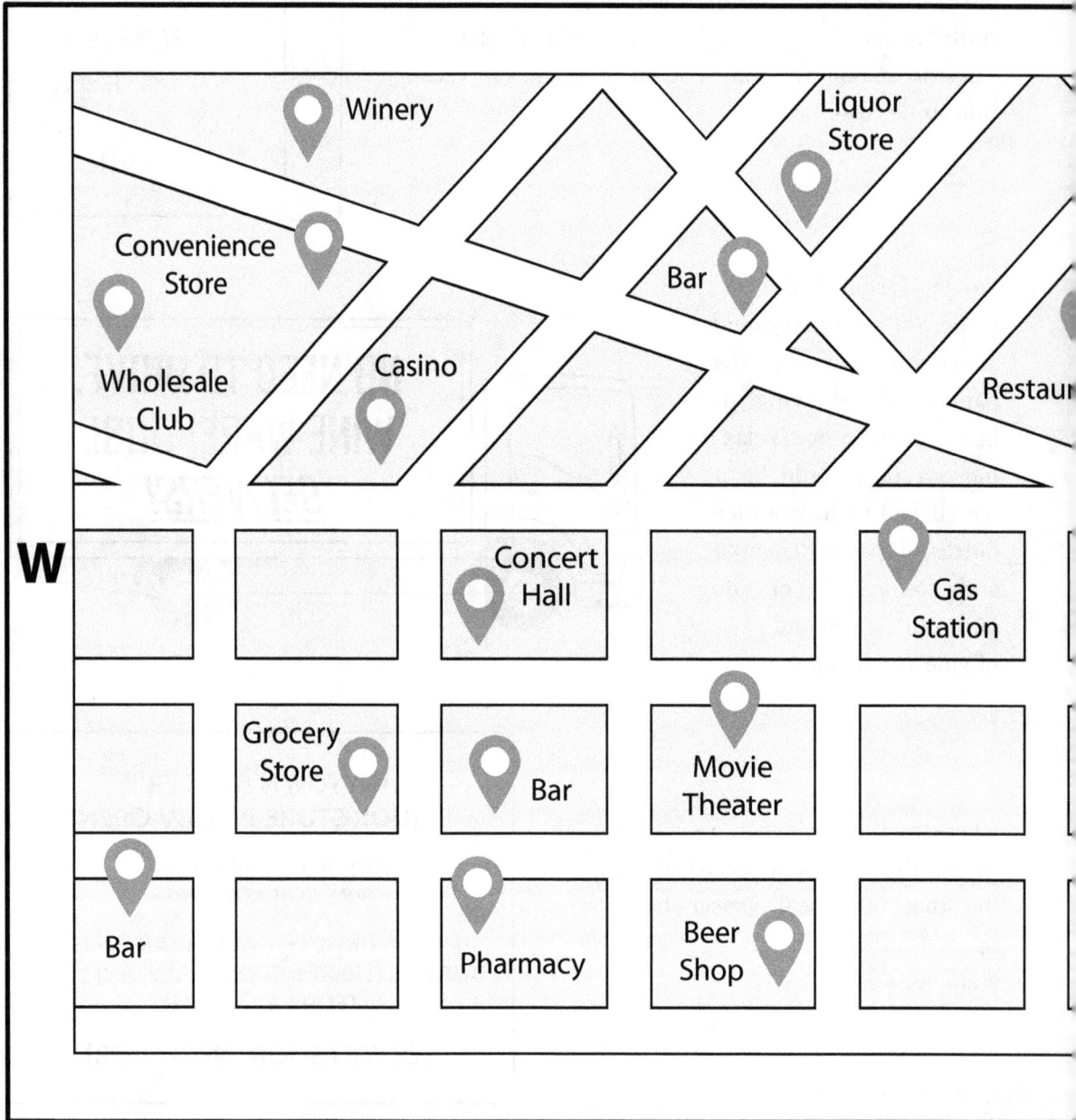

Winery

Liquor Store

Convenience Store

Bar

Wholesale Club

Casino

Restaur

W

Concert Hall

Gas Station

Grocery Store

Bar

Movie Theater

Bar

Pharmacy

Beer Shop

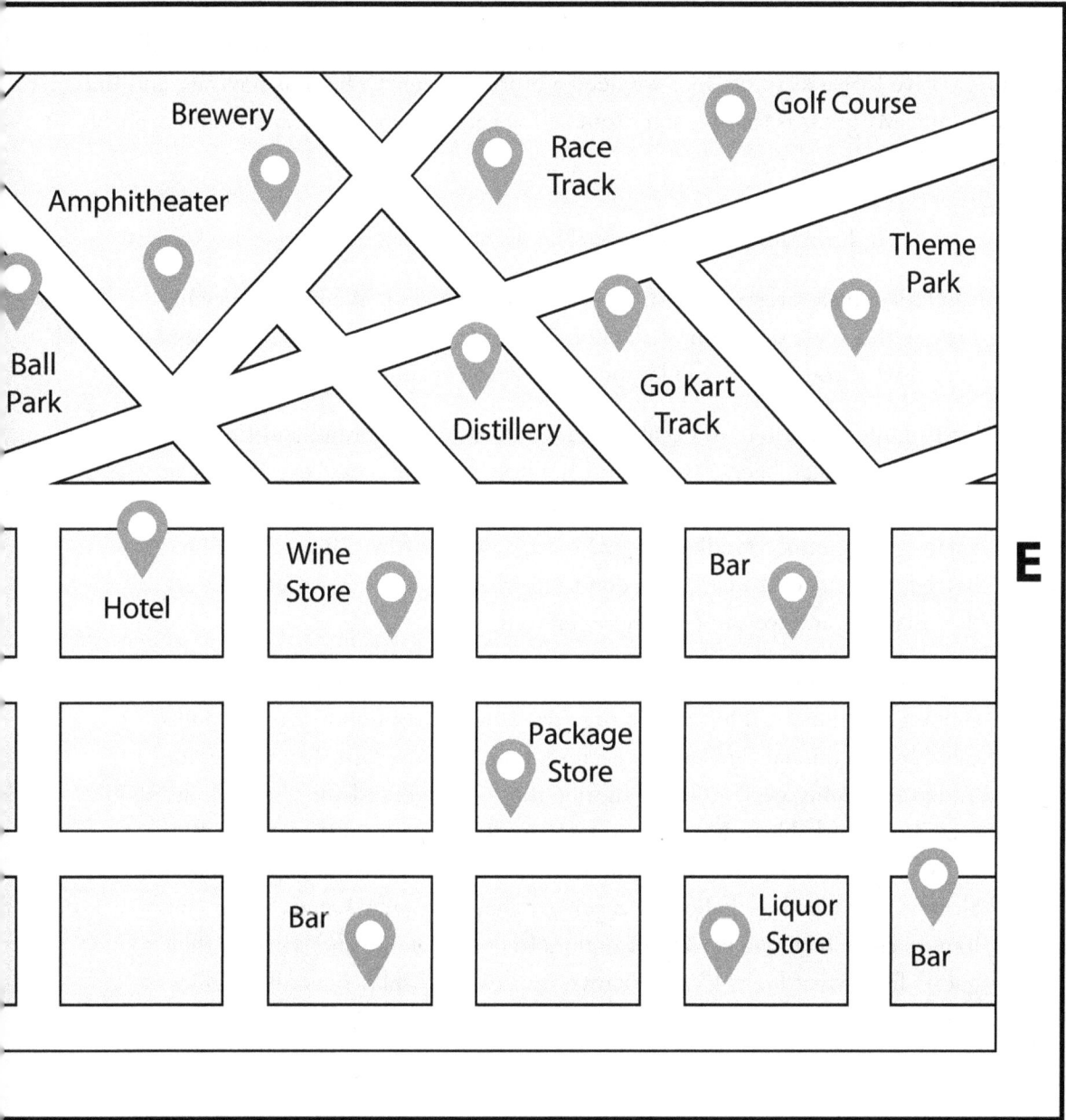

alcohol near me

Brewery

Golf Course

Amphitheater

Race
Track

Theme
Park

Ball
Park

Distillery

Go Kart
Track

E

Hotel

Wine
Store

Bar

Package
Store

Bar

Liquor
Store

Bar

# The Most Effective Product Packaging on the Planet

The packaging for all of the types, flavors and brands of alcohol have become so alluring and competitive that it's almost like we need a Store Greeter to help us navigate and find what we want. My guess is that person's tour of the retail liquor landscape would probably sound like this:

> Hi, I'm Daniel. Welcome to The Alcohol Store.
>
> You look a little overwhelmed. This is understandable. We have a very big store with a wide selection of alcohol. However, you'll see how simple it is to find what you want if you let me to show you around.
>
> First of all, let me tell you that we carry almost every brand and flavor of the most popular beers, wines and liquors. And we stock everything in just about every imaginable size: Kegs, Cases, 12-Packs, 6-Packs, Tall Boys, Forties, Magnums, Handles, Jugs, Boxes, Liters, Fifths, Pints, Half Pints, Bottles, Cans and Minis. If you don't see what you want here, chances are they make it, and we can get it here for you!
>
> Now, if you'll turn your attention to the right side of the store, these aisles contain our liquors. This area is organized by the six liquor types as indicated by directional signs above each section: Brandy, Gin, Rum, Tequila, Vodka and Whiskey. You'll also notice the various brands on the shelf are each distinguishable by a special and unique-looking appearance: Clear Bottle, Colored Bottle, Etched Bottle . . . Tall Shapes, Skinny Shapes, Curvy Shapes . . . Cowboy Labels, Recycled Labels, Foreign Labels. Our customers enjoy buying a variety of liquors to have at home and serve to their guests from what looks like their own impressive display of adult trophies. Fun, right?!

On our left are the wine aisles. We display our wine inventory according to the five types: Red, White, Rose, Sparkling and Dessert. And because the appearance of the important-looking bottles and fancy labels are all very similar, we recommend you join our wine of the week club to learn what you like. It's a subscription plan that delivers new wines right to your door without you having to worry about running out of alcohol or forgetting which ones you want to buy again for your own sophisticated wine rack display at home. Easy, right?!

Here along the entire center of the store, we have our display of alcohol gift sets. These decorative packages include one bottle of your favorite liquor and two glasses. They're perfect to bring to a holiday gathering or dinner party. And they're really great as a housewarming present to friends who just moved in to their new place but haven't unpacked their glasses yet. If you wanna see smiles as soon as they open their front door, just bring them one of these alcohol gift sets. Generous, right?!

At the rear of the store is our open cooler display of ice cold foreign, domestic and micro-brewery beers. Beer is a versatile choice because it is enjoyed equally by casual drinkers straight from the container, or by more sophisticated drinkers who believe it tastes better when poured into a special glass or mug. Oh, and our section of beer in cans is right over here. Cans are the right choice for pool parties and barefoot barbeques. You don't want to be the cause of a bloody foot from a dropped beer bottle after the joint starts jumpin'. Thoughtful, right?!

Take a look around, and if you have any questions, come see me at the front of the store. I'll be greeting the constant stream of customers as they come in and directing them to the shortest line at our registers when they're ready to check out.

Oh, and by the way, the front of the store is also where we have our travel liquors. You know, the plastic liquor bottles that fit safely in your shoulder bag or backpack when you wanna drink while you're on the go. Smart, right?!

Have a great visit! "

# The Most Brilliant Tagline of All Time

The following is an extremely condensed conversation based on a story that's *probably true:*

**Advertising Creative Director (ACD):** *Hey. Great news. We just landed a new account. The client is a special interest coalition formed by all the alcohol manufacturers, distributors and retailers around the world.*

**Advertising Creative Writer (ACW):** *Whoa. Very cool. What do they want us to do?*

**ACD:** *They want us to come up with a sort of public service announcement in the form of a product tagline that will appear with every alcohol advertisement on the planet from now on.*

**ACW:** *Whoa—WOW. That's a tall order, Boss. Has to be meaningful to every level of their sell chain as well as understandable to every man, woman and child. AND simple enough to be translated into every language.*

**ACD:** *Exactly. They want this tagline to restore people's confident enjoyment of alcohol while responding to the negative messages people constantly see and hear about the common danger of drunk driving and the rising number of alcohol rehabs. And here's the kicker. This tagline has to check three boxes: Instructions, Warning and Disclaimer.*

**ACW:** *Geeeeeeeezzzz, Boss! You're asking me to spin straw into gold!*

**ACD:** *Yup. But we're going to come up with it together. So let's get to work.*

**ACW:** *Alright. So if we start with the instructions piece, I think people need to know that drinking alcohol is enjoyable because it helps you feel relaxed and have more fun.*

**ACD:** *Yes. And if we roll-in the warning part, alcohol is legal for adults, not kids. And when you drink you have to pace yourself and be responsible not to have too much, or else you'll impair your judgment or get sick, or both.*

ACW: *That's IT!*

ACD: *What's it?*

ACW: *Drink Responsibly!*

ACD: *Okay. Good instructions. Warning is in there too. But how does it also communicate the disclaimer?*

ACW: *Think about it. By including the words 'Drink Responsibly' at the end of every alcohol ad, the alcohol companies are reminding everyone, 'Yeah, we showed you images of fun and relaxed people with our product. We also inferred that they're drinking it responsibly. So don't blame us if you had a different experience with our product, because that's your fault, not ours.'*

ACD: *HO-LEE-COW! This is brilliant! Drink Responsibly! Instructions, Warning and Disclaimer all rolled into one powerfully-clear two-word product tagline!*

ACW: *Yeah, and it also answers people's questions about the possible consequences of alcohol. Under-age drinking? . . . that's not responsible. Drunk driving? . . . not a responsible choice either. Drinking made you sick? . . . well, that doesn't match the responsible drinking people we advertise. Drinking made you go to rehab? . . . then, you must have not been drinking responsibly.*

ACD: *Perfect. So, what the alcohol companies will basically be saying when they add 'Drink Responsibly' to all of their marketing materials is: 'Good drinking experience? . . . We're responsible. Bad drinking experience? . . . You're responsible.'*

ACW: *Right on, Boss. Clean hands for our client, and a heads-up for their customers. Mission accomplished.*

# THE FINE PRINT
# THAT ISN'T PRINTED

Mind Altering

Habit Forming

Stomach Irritating

Affects Everyone Differently

Difficult To Gauge The Influence

*. . . because reading is a buzzkill*

# Alcohol is a Mind-Altering Substance

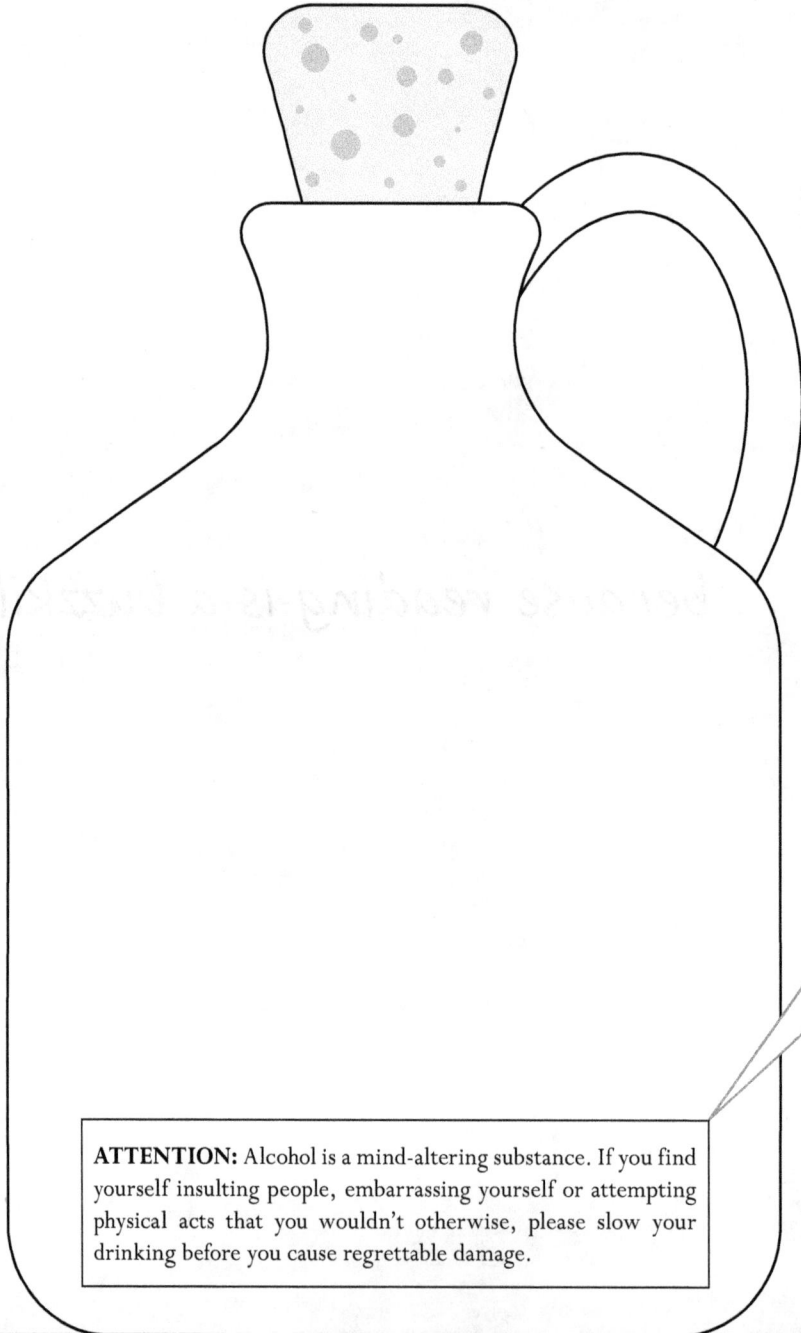

**ATTENTION:** Alcohol is a mind-altering substance. If you find yourself insulting people, embarrassing yourself or attempting physical acts that you wouldn't otherwise, please slow your drinking before you cause regrettable damage.

**ATTENTION:** Alcohol is a mind-altering substance. If you find yourself insulting people, embarrassing yourself or attempting physical acts that you wouldn't otherwise, please slow your drinking before you cause regrettable damage.

# Alcohol is a Habit-Forming Substance

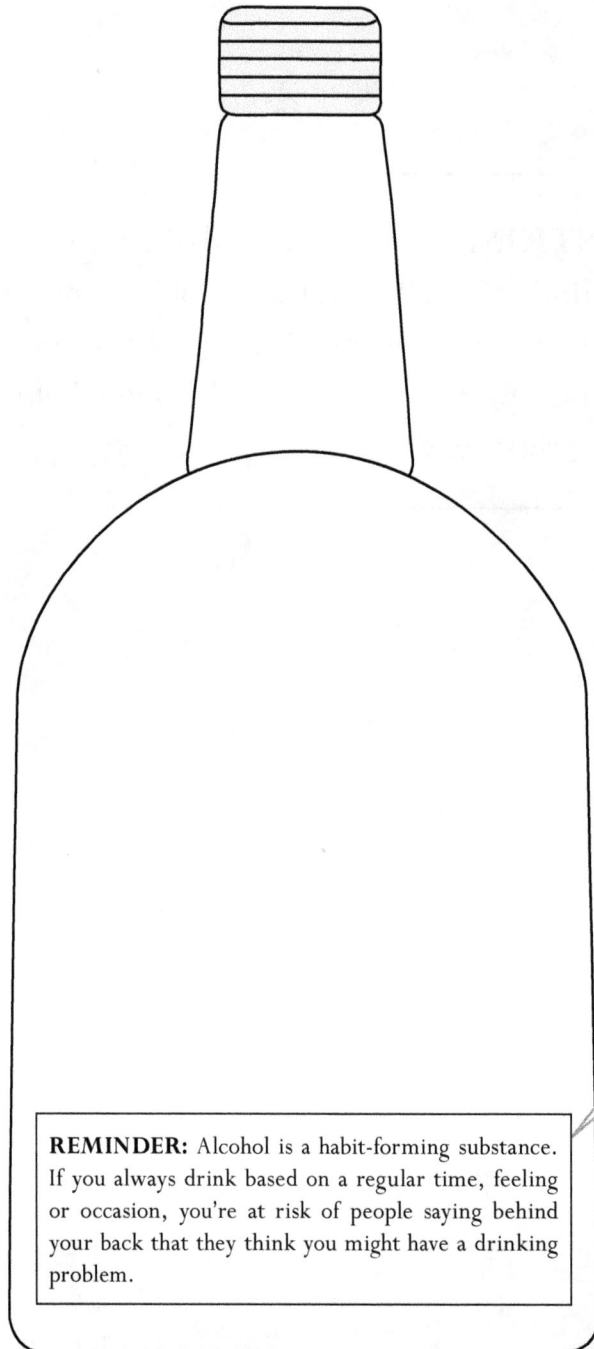

**REMINDER:** Alcohol is a habit-forming substance. If you always drink based on a regular time, feeling or occasion, you're at risk of people saying behind your back that they think you might have a drinking problem.

**REMINDER:** Alcohol is a habit-forming substance. If you always drink based on a regular time, feeling or occasion, you're at risk of people saying behind your back that they think you might have a drinking problem.

# Alcohol is a Stomach Irritant

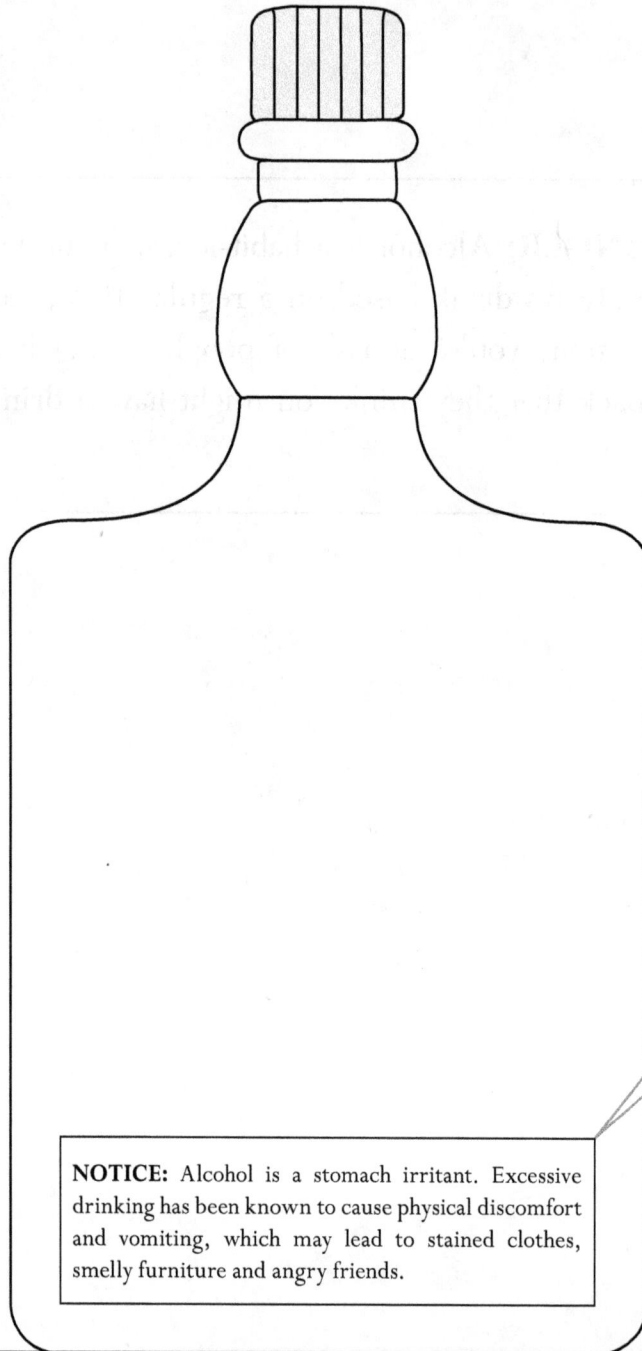

**NOTICE:** Alcohol is a stomach irritant. Excessive drinking has been known to cause physical discomfort and vomiting, which may lead to stained clothes, smelly furniture and angry friends.

**NOTICE:** Alcohol is a stomach irritant. Excessive drinking has been known to cause physical discomfort and vomiting, which may lead to stained clothes, smelly furniture and angry friends.

# Alcohol Affects Everyone Differently

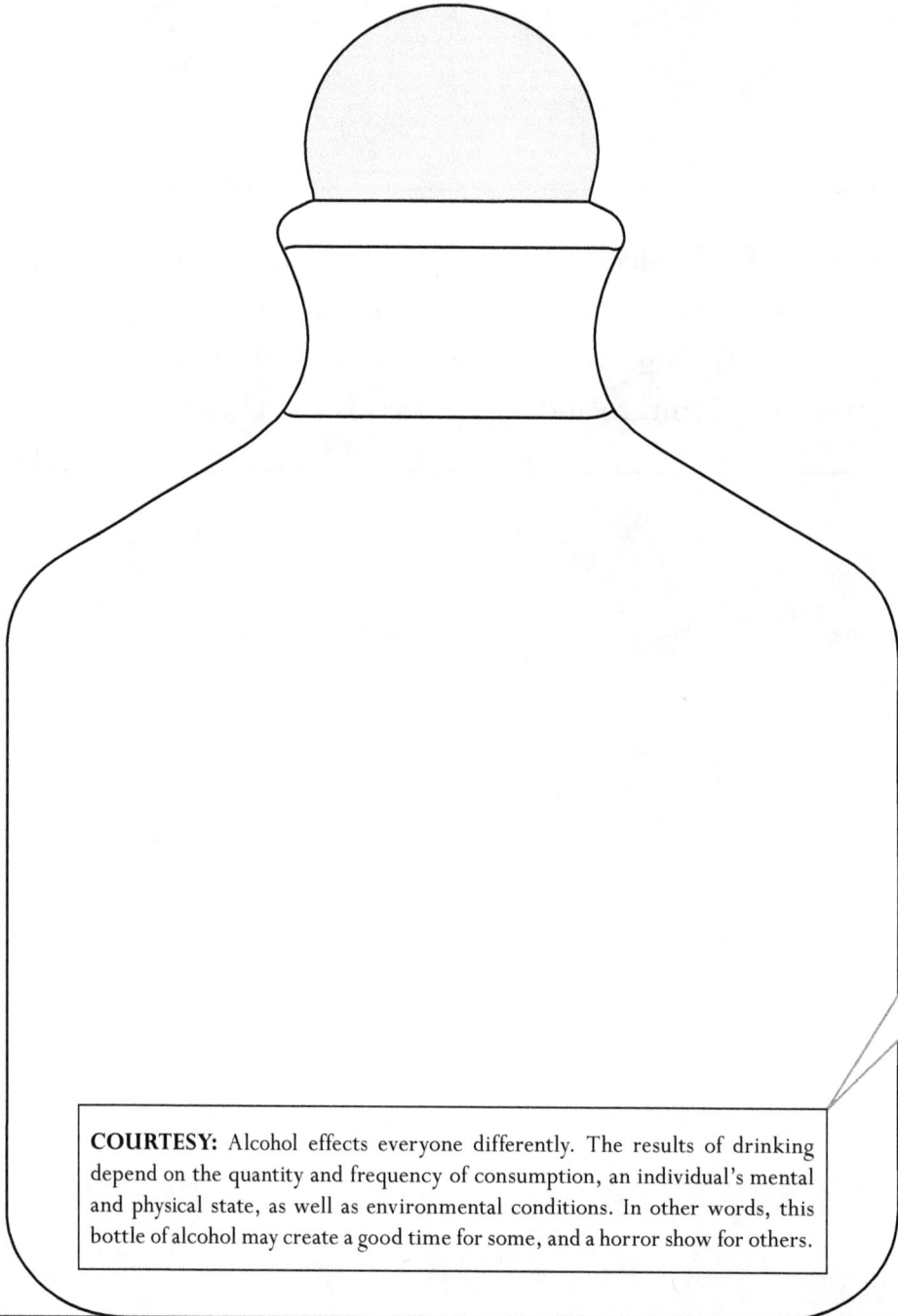

**COURTESY:** Alcohol effects everyone differently. The results of drinking depend on the quantity and frequency of consumption, an individual's mental and physical state, as well as environmental conditions. In other words, this bottle of alcohol may create a good time for some, and a horror show for others.

**COURTESY:** Alcohol effects everyone differently. The results of drinking depend on the quantity and frequency of consumption, an individual's mental and physical state, as well as environmental conditions. In other words, this bottle of alcohol may create a good time for some, and a horror show for others.

# The Influence of Alcohol is Difficult to Gauge

**TIP:** The influence of alcohol is difficult to gauge. When you repeatedly say 'Last One' but continue to have more drinks, you may already be headin for trouble.

**TIP:** The influence of alcohol is difficult to gauge. When you repeatedly say 'Last One' but continue to have more drinks, you may already be headin for trouble.

# THE SIDE EFFECTS THAT AREN'T DISCUSSED

Mysterious Stains, Scratches, Breaks, Bruises & Burns

Missing Keys, Glasses, Shoe, Phone & Underwear

Undesirable Tattoos, Bar Bills & Sexcapades

Tired Homecare, Hobbies & Reflections

Stalled Careers & Relationships

. . . because it's not embarrassing
if we can avoid talking about it

# Mysterious Stains, Scratches, Breaks, Bruises & Burns

During our more reckless times consuming alcohol, when our mind and body have finally had enough, we just pass out wherever we are at that moment. However, with a little drinking practice, we learn to predict the arrival of this personal shut-down event, and we make it home safe just in time to collapse and sleep it off in peace. Additionally, this pass-out-at-home practice also yields us damage-control-from-home practice. So after we come-to alone in the safety of our own homes enough times, we learn that the damage that resulted from our drinking doesn't have to be embarrassing as long as we use the avoidance tactic: Hiding The Evidence.

Opening our eyes to see a brown stain on the seat of our new white jeans laying next to us on the coffee table could be terribly embarrassing. But if none of our friends call with an awful story about how we got so drunk that we soiled ourselves, it's not that bad. We can just buy another pair of jeans and hope our pooping problem wasn't a public event.
*(Hiding Tactic: Don't ask, don't tell.)*

Getting up from the couch to see the scratched leather couch cushion on the floor that we somehow damaged the last time we got this drunk is not a pleasant reminder. The good news is, we can just turn the cushion back over again, put it back on the couch, and go back to pretending there are no scratches on our gorgeous leather couch.
*(Hiding Tactic: Outta sight, outta mind.)*

Making it to the bathroom mirror to find out what's causing the searing pain we feel on our face, we see the raised blue bruise in the center of our forehead and broken toilet lid half falling into the tank. But because we didn't knock our front teeth out, we can just wear a hat the next few days, replace a toilet tank lid, and no one has to know about the break or the bruise.
*(Hiding Tactic: Almost a problem isn't a problem.)*

Smelling some kind of burnt food odor hanging in the house, we glide along the wall until we arrive at the stove where we are stunned but relieved to see that we must have passed out while heating up leftovers that have been burnt to charcoal in the bottom of a pot. No harm done though, because we can easily trash the burnt pot, and just open the windows to air-out the smell without anyone ever knowing we almost burned the place down.

*(Hiding Tactic: Place needed to be cleaned anyway.)*

# Missing Keys, Glasses, Shoe, Phone & Underwear

Sometimes after a long session of drinking, and after our mind starts to clear up, we realize that one or more of the things we brought out with us did not return home with us. This can be frustrating. Especially if it isn't the first time this has happened. However, we also know from our past experiences that losing our things doesn't have to be embarrassing—as long as we're careful to avoid telling anyone that we did it *again*.

---

### Avoidance Tactic: Controlling the Conversation

**Saying:**

*"Hey Sis! Great idea to ride together, right?! This way we get some one-on-one time together before we get to Mom and Dad's Sunday barbeque. So good to see you! What's new?!"*

**Thinking:**

*". . . gotta get another set of keys made again. The only way I was even able to get inside this morning was to use the housekey I hid outside after the last time I drank all night, lost my keys and had to call my sister for help."*

---

### Avoidance Tactic: Side-Stepping the Question

**Saying:**

*"These are prescription sunglasses, Mom. I wore 'em because I knew we'd all be visiting and eating outside in this gorgeous weather! You should put your sunglasses on too, Mom. The bright sun is not good for your eyes either."*

**Thinking:**

*". . . not sure why I took off my regular glasses or where I left 'em while I was out drinking last night, because I can't see a thing without 'em. But, thank God for next day shipping. Maybe I should have ordered two pairs?"*

## Avoidance Tactic: Changing the Subject

**Saying:** "Of course I'm gonna return your pink stilettos. This week, okay? Oh, and I'm also going to let you borrow my new riding boots. When was the last time you went riding?"

**Thinking:** "... as soon as I buy you a new pair of pink stilettos and scrape up the bottoms a little so you don't know I got so drunk Friday night that I lost one. Still beyond even my imagination how I managed to get home with only one shoe."

## Avoidance Tactic: Diverting the Attention

**Saying:** "Yes, everything's really good, Uncle Ed. But, hold that thought. Just gotta text Sherry back and let her know I'll call her later. Okay. Done. Thanks. Yes, work is great! Friends are great! Everything's great!"

**Thinking:** "... and I'm so smart! All I have to do is wait for everyone else to text me too, then add their name to the number that comes in, and nobody has to know that I got so drunk again that I had to replace another lost phone."

## Avoidance Tactic: Good Things in Common

**Saying:** "Oh, I didn't realize anyone would notice I'm not wearing a bra. Thank you so much for the down-low compliment though, Gramma Dee. I think you look amazing too! Great genes are such a blessing in our family, huh?!"

**Thinking:** "...don't think Gramma Dee would be as complimentary if she knew I wasn't wearing any panties either. Definitely gotta stop getting so wasted that I keep misplacing my underwear around town."

# Undesirable Tattoos, Bar Bills & Sexcapades

Arriving back at work the next morning, it's always fun to hear and share a good story about the previous night's happy hour or weekend drink-fest. And with some experience telling drinking stories that bore or scare people, we learn how to tell them the right way. It has to be safe, but still a little reckless. A little reckless, but still have a happy ending. And above all else, the whole drinking story has to be honest, but A-D-D brief. The Avoidance Tactic that we use to talk around the embarrassing parts of our alcohol outings while recapping the fun parts is called, telling 'Half-Truths.'

So when we see Conservative Ken walk into work Monday morning with a wry smile on his face and a bandage showing thru his shirt, naturally, we wanna know what happened with his buddies from out of town.

Or when we see Livin' Large Leo giving his always entertaining Monday morning extravagant party weekend recap for everyone getting their first cup from the department coffee machine, we hear his past weekend was extra-large because he was trying to impress his little brother into going back to finish his college degree, so he can live large like Leo too.

Or when Only-Wine-Wendy arrives at work, we all want to know what happened since she stunned us the night before by doing tequila shots, kissing Partytime Penny, and then leaving the bar with Fun Frank.

And we all know that Ken, Leo and Wendy probably left out the uncomfortable parts of their stories, but no one wants to hear about those anyway.

So when we walk in on Conservative Ken shaking his head in the office men's room mirror looking at his tattoo of large black eyelashes around his left nipple, we exit before he sees us and keep it to ourselves—just like we'd want someone to do if they saw the huge handcuffs tattooed across both of our cheeks that we keep outta sight.

And when we overhear Livin' Large Leo on a desperate call to increase his credit line, we silently wish him luck and thank our lucky stars that we found a roommate situation because of our already wrecked credit.

The best is when the fun but uncomfortable part of the drunken story that someone half-truth-tells about is US. Like when we're Fun Frank's new roommate that nobody knows about. And we happen to be in the right place at the right time when he got home with Only-Wine-Wendy. And upon seeing both of us, Wendy decided she didn't just want a one-night stand. Wendy wanted a threesome.

"I finally got a tattoo! Cool, right?! We decided to do the bar crawl around stadium places all day Saturday. Never been—loved it! The game was awesome, until the end, so we went drinkin some more after the game. I really thought I would win that bet I made. Anyway, my buddies encouraged me to get a tattoo on my chest. So I finally did it. Hurt like hell. I'd show you guys, but I gotta keep it bandaged for a while. Gotta get to work. Catch up with you guys later."

"Mannn . . . first my brother and I met up with my Crew in the V-I-P at Poone for bottle service 'til midnight. Then we partied at The Waterbleau nightclub, crashed in the suite I bought for the night, and Sunday we all hung by the Waterbleau pool in a full-bar service cabana I reserved for the next day. And that's how you live on the weekends, Leo Style! Gotta make a couple calls. See you fellas at lunch later!"

"Oh, everybody has to let loose once in a while. So I kissed a girl. So I had a one night stand. So what. Frank and I are both consenting adults, and we had a glorious evening of drunken sex all around his place—couch, kitchen, shower, his bed, his new roommate's bed. Hope you guys have a great day too. Gotta get to work. Talk to y'all later."

# Tired Homecare, Hobbies & Reflections

The drinking lifestyle is fun. Because everybody drinks. And because we all enjoy socializing. So it makes sense that not long after we turn 21, we begin to fall into the same social lifestyle pattern as most adults: drinking while socializing as a calendared activity. Whether our drinking is an accessory activity to the primary get-together—like Wednesday night bowling and Saturday afternoon golf. Or when drinking is the primary activity—like Friday night happy hour or Sunday late-morning brunch. All these drinking occasions are fine, and normal, and safe, and pretty much expected – which is fine with us too. So no one really thinks twice that we're drinking four times a week, because no one's drinking excessively or hurting themselves or hurting others—as far as we know. And as long we only spend time with people who are also living the same work-life balance with alcohol, we have no idea of the tired side effects that are slowly increasing along with the frequency of our lifestyle drinking.

But when an old friend or distant family member comes to visit us who doesn't drink as much or as often, the side effects are apparent to them whether we choose to see the evidence also or not.

This Avoidance Tactic is called: '*Yes, but*', and usually sounds a lot like this:

> Oh my goodness! Come in! I'm so glad you're here! Welcome to my first home that I actually own!

Just leave your bags here for now and let me show you around.

It's been so long. I can tell you're as fit as ever. Yes, I know I'm fat, but I'm happy!

Come with me to the kitchen. I have beer and wine in the fridge, liquor here on the counter, and the vodka is in the freezer, of course! Obviously, I'm having a drink, so what can I get for you? Nothing yet?! Okay, I'll finish showing you around, but then I'm gonna make you something so we can sit and sip while we catch up!

Oh, and before I forget, when you turn the kitchen faucet on, just leave that big plastic bowl over the handle. It works fine as long as you keep the bowl in place to catch the spray. Don't worry, I have friends over all the time using it, and the water just drains into the sink, so they don't even notice the bowl anymore. Yes, it's a little awkward to use the faucet the first couple times, but I just haven't had any free time to get it fixed!

Okay, now bring your bags and come this way and I'll show you to the guest room I created.

As you can see, I set it up for triple-use as my guest room, home theater and gaming room. The huge screen and surround sound are great for having friends over for drinks and gaming parties. It's also awesome for Sunday afternoon binge watching TV shows in bed and recovering from all the weekend alcohol before work starts again Monday morning! Yes, I know watching screens is not a real hobby, but it's a smart layout, right?!

The door on the left is the guest bathroom. Everything works in there! Except there's no full-length mirror. Not that you need it—you still look amazing! I just haven't hung any of my mirrors up yet. You know, until I get myself lookin' good again. No need to depress myself with mirrors all over my house, right?! But I'll get around to it eventually!

You know what? Instead of staying in, let's go down to the pub! I wanna introduce you to my friends. They're so nice and relaxed and fun. Just leave all your things here. We'll all be back here tonight anyway. You're gonna love everybody!

Let's go right now! 🙶

# Stalled Careers & Relationships

Everyone's on social media because it's the most fun and easy way to share and catch up with friends and family.

However, the more frequently we make drinking alcohol a part of our work-life balance, the more it influences our thinking and choices, which also influences our social media updates. So the more often we drink, the less we realize that our posts are also being read by some of our friends and family who are concerned about our interpretation of feel-good relationships, activities and accomplishments.

Unlike the previously described avoidance tactics in this section that are all consciously executed, this one is different. This one is the result of drinking more quantities at more occasions among people who also drink and post similar alcohol-related updates. This avoidance tactic is subconscious. And it's a little scary to those who love us, want the best for us, and wonder why we don't see that our life perspective is getting way off course. This type of avoidance is called alcohol-induced delusion.

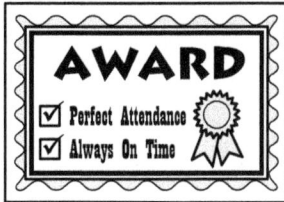

Sales and Innovation Awards are great but showing up on time every day is even more important! I'm for sure on my way to running this biz one day! But today I'm on my way to HAPPY HOUR!

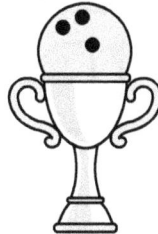

Getting the league sportsmanship trophy is proof that drinkin and socializin does make you a winner! Congrats to all my friends on our Wrecked Crew bowling team! Last place score but 1st place hearts!

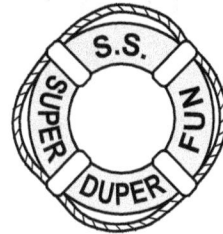

So many positives with a romantic couples cruise va-cay y'all . . . one price room, food, drinks . . . cruise drinkin with other fun couples is like an adult dorm party . . . what happens on a cruise stays on a cruise!

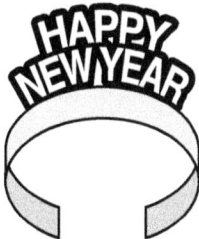

Me and my friends have the same new year resolution every year . . . just party bigger and better than last year . . . and we did it again! Here's to US . . . livin' life like it should be lived!

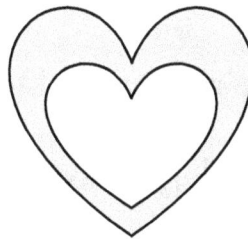

Our drunk party pass out sex life is THE BEST! Especially when it happens on my MOST FAVORITE HOLIDAY! Love you, BOO BOO!

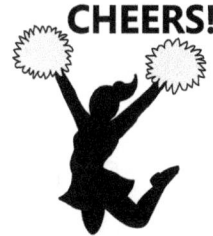

OMG 5 years at the same job! My first promotion and pay raise must be next, RIGHT?! I know it's only Tuesday but I'll be at the bar after work if y'all wanna join . . . CHEERS!

# THE INFLUENCE THAT EVERYONE'S UNDER

Whether We're Having Drinks or Not

Every Age, Gender, Lifestyle and Location

More Powerful Than Paid Advertisements

As Normal as Clean Clothes & Fresh Breath

Even With Eyes-Wide-Open, Seeing is Still a Choice

*. . . because alcohol marketing*
*is better than we realize*

# Whether We're Having Drinks or Not

Okay, so we've arrived at the cherry-on-top summary section of this story about alcohol.

Remember I told you near the beginning that you'd enjoy the ride? Been fun—right?! And isn't it amazing how we all recognize the circumstances and quotes about alcohol as if they could have been us or happened around us?!

Well, there's a really good reason all of us have very similar alcohol experiences, understandings and tendencies.

Simply put, we have been taught to *believe* the same handful of things about alcohol and drinking responsibly are all we need to know. So when we hear about or encounter something about alcohol, our minds automatically understand it based on the following seven filters:

One, we all *believe* we know *what* alcohol is . . . it's a safe and widely available product that comes in many flavors and appearances for adults to choose to drink while socializing.

Two, we all *believe* we know *why* adults drink alcohol . . . it's a quick, easy and civilized way to feel relaxed or have a fun experience.

Three, we all *believe* we know *when* adults drink alcohol . . . it's acceptable at any time of day and occasion except when driving, pregnant or breastfeeding.

Four, we all *believe* we know *where* adults drink alcohol . . . it's acceptable everywhere except in working, learning or exercising environments.

Five, we all *believe* we know *how* adults drink alcohol . . . it's acceptable in any amount and frequency without becoming sick, falling asleep or slurring.

Six, we all *believe* that any choices with alcohol or consequences because of alcohol that are beyond what we consider socially acceptable are simply the result of not drinking responsibly.

Seven, we all *believe* that while not drinking responsibly is not acceptable, we tolerate and forgive as long as the person is sorry and can control themselves to drink responsibly more often than not.

And so, now that we're all aware that it's the same limited beliefs we've been taught that make all of us under the influence of alcohol—whether we're drinking or not—it's time to move on to the unlimited part of this cherry-on-top summary section.

# Every Age, Gender, Lifestyle and Location

That's right, I'm sayin' that everyone everywhere is under the influence of alcohol.

Think about it. The messages about alcohol that we hear and believe and relay to each other reach all of us indiscriminately, no matter where we are on the planet.

Ask any kid under the age of 21 about alcohol, and every one of them will not only know what it is, they will also answer from the same set of limited beliefs as everyone over the age of 21: *My Mommy likes wine after a hard day . . . My Daddy is sorry he has to take us to the playground later because he drank too much last night . . . I love weddings because all the adults drink and then wanna have fun dancing with me! . . . When I'm 21, I'm not gonna smoke but I'm gonna drink!*

Listen to any male or female exchange about what someone is drinking and why, and every one of them will prove how gender-neutral our alcohol choices have become: *Look, she's drinking a beer, that means she's causal and approachable . . . His glass of wine means he's calm and classy . . . Her martini means she's strong and sophisticated . . . His mimosa in a champagne flute means he's secure and stylish.*

Watch any gathering of people who have an obvious lifestyle preference, and every one of their venues will have alcohol available while they socialize . . . Democratic Conventions, Republican Rallies, LGBTQ Parades, Business Networking, Car Shows, Sporting Events, (you get the idea).

Imagine any remote location on the planet where people live: jungles, glaciers, forests, deserts. If a traveler has ever passed through and shared his alcohol with any of the locals, chances are the local store now stocks alcohol for sale. And if the local population is more than just a few people, that local store probably also has a bar attached to it (wink).

So now that we all agree that we're all under the influence of alcohol—every age, gender and lifestyle in every location on earth—whether we're drinking or not. Let's keep moving on and take a look at how alcohol advertising contributes to this worldwide influence.

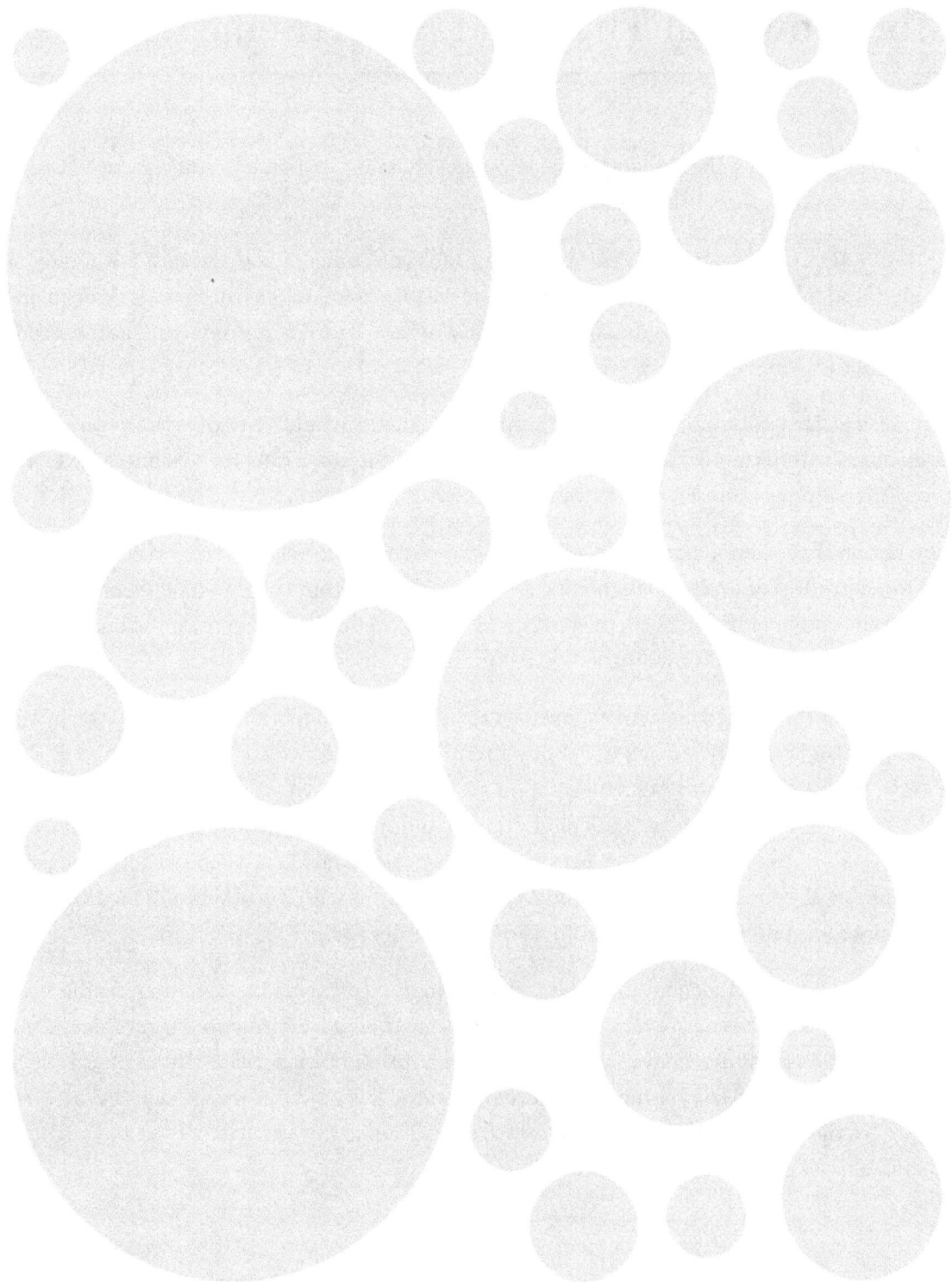

# More Powerful Than Paid Advertisements

Yes, at the end of the previous page, I purposely said *'contributes'*—rather than *'causes'* this worldwide alcohol influence.

I know you probably read the foreshadowing table of contents and thought I was gonna blame the alcohol companies for our sometimes not-so-good experiences with their product. But I'm not gonna make that point, nor do I believe that it's entirely true. Partly true, yeah—but to completely blame them, nah.

The answer is simple, but it's not *that* simple. Besides, I wouldn't have written an entire book about rethinking drinking just to connect all of the story dots for you and arrive at a thoughtless finger-pointing explanation like *blame*.

The reason that alcohol marketing is better than we realize is because every day we receive the same handful of limited belief messages about alcohol from three independent sources. And even though only one of them is paid advertising, they all collaborate and complement each other in subtle but powerful ways to put all of us under the influence.

Let's start with the paid advertising messages. Just like any big brand soda, water or juice, alcohol is also creatively pitched to get our attention wherever we are. During our everyday travels, we hear refreshing beer tops popping on our radios, we see billboard-size celebrities giving their endorsement of alcohol brands, and we pass countless retail signs letting us know which shops have liquor, beer or wine for sale. And then when we get home, it's the same background hum of alcohol advertising mixed-in with the other safe, civilized and social products and services pitched to us on our family room TVs.

The second source of alcohol messaging is viral marketing. This has always been the holy grail of marketing, because every business aspires for their advertising to trigger sales AND spur ongoing consumer conversations about their product or service that create EVEN MORE SALES. Very few businesses have achieved the level of viral acceptance that alcohol has where the product or service is not only freely discussed, it's also expected and encouraged in almost every social situation.

The third is entertainment placement. Because we so commonly include alcohol at our barbeques, birthdays, brunches and every occasion in between, it makes perfect sense that many of our favorite TV shows, movies and songs also include alcohol. However, our entertainers are not intentionally selling us alcohol; they're just using alcohol to make their characters and storylines come off as more relatable to us. Think about it: alcohol companies don't need to pay to show their labels or mention specific brands for us to understand the role it's playing in TV and movie scenes. We sing along just as loud without needing to know what kind of tequila makes her clothes fall off. None of us needs to be told what's in the tall slender-brown bottle that the lovable TV Parent grabs from the family fridge after work. And all of us know what's in the very fancy glass that the admirable Movie Hero is drinking while relaxing in between very important pursuits.

Let me drive the point home with some numbers about the effect of these three converging message sources. If your business could spend 25 cents on advertising to make 1 dollar in revenue, it stands to reason that you'd spend 250 million to make 1 billion, right? Well, the alcohol industry as a whole currently spends between 2–3 billion a year on worldwide advertising to make about 1.5 trillion in revenue, while just the non-alcohol beverage company Coca-Cola currently spends 3.8 billion on worldwide advertising to make 32 billion in revenue[*].

I know . . . the numbers are just jaw-dropping, right?!

It's almost like alcohol marketing is beyond viral . . . is there anything *bigger* than viral marketing?!

The bottom-line here is that although it's the huge amount of money that the alcohol industry spends in advertising that kicks off our awareness of their product, it's our social conversations and popular entertainment that drives alcohol product sales so much higher than non-alcohol products AND makes the influence of alcohol feel like a normal part of our everyday experience, whether we choose to drink or not.

---

[*] "Advertising and the Alcohol Industry," Encyclopedia.com, March 31, 2020, https://www.encyclopedia.com/education/encyclopedias-almanacs-transcripts-and-maps/advertising-and-alcohol-industry

"Alcoholic Drinks," Statista, 2020, https://www.statista.com/outlook/10000000/100/alcoholic-drinks/worldwide

"Coca-Cola Company's advertising expense from 2014 to 2019," Statista, March 2, 2020, https://www.statista.com/statistics/286526/coca-cola-advertising-spending-worldwide/

# As Normal as Clean Clothes and Fresh Breath

Okay, let's wrap up this summary section.

Remember at the beginning of this story we talked about my neighbor Lorenzo getting dropped off by police at his house next door because he got drunk and lost his phone and car and wallet?

And you remember all of that prompted my son to get really excited and call Lorenzo an idiot, so I set out to try and understand what's really goin' on with our relationship with alcohol because I wanted to be able to explain to my son why some people can't seem to drink responsibly?

Well, now that I've explained throughout out this book the journey of how we all grew up with alcohol, and most of us have good experiences with alcohol, and all us of have at least been around when someone has a not-so-good experience with alcohol, and that all of us are under the influence of alcohol whether we're drinking or not . . . it's time to tell you my *Ah-Ha* about it all.

Since our childhoods, we've all been on a steady diet of the three-way source of alcohol messaging that I mentioned in the previous chapter (advertising/conversations/entertainment). What it's done is convince us that alcohol consumption is *normal* . . . that getting tipsy is *normal* . . . that making a mess with their product isn't pleasant and our fault—but it's *normal* too. That's right, we honestly believe that drinking socially is as normal as showing up to the social occasion with clean clothes and fresh breath. We buy laundry detergent and toothpaste to feel clean while socializing, and we buy alcohol to feel relaxed while socializing.

And why has it been so easy to sell us on the belief that an arguably unnecessary product is a household staple? Because it works: it delivers the easy smiles and harmless fun depicted in the advertising and in our favorite movies, TV shows and songs. Sometimes we actually like feeling better without doing better. Because sometimes doing better is hard, and because sometimes adults just want the feeling of getting a trophy.

And that's all alcohol is. It's a relief, a solution, a celebration, a reward—whether we earned it or not. And simply wanting more of that feeling is what makes alcohol so slippery for many of us.

So, what happened with Lorenzo? He just likes to feel relaxed, so he drinks too much sometimes. Is he drinking to feel so relaxed that he forgets to solve some life problem? Maybe. Or, is his attraction to alcohol like loving peanuts but being allergic to them? Maybe. Either way, should he rethink of his current circumstance as normal, and start believing that alcohol is keeping him from the true solution he's trying to feel? I think so.

And what about Camilla? Well, she also just wants to believe her husband is normal. So she tolerates his iterations of trying to drink alcohol like a normal person. Because the alternative she's been taught is too unpleasant: that her husband *isn't normal*. So, should she rethink a little about what's normal, and that maybe instead of tolerating her husband continuing to make messes while trying to drink responsibly, she should make herself open and available to a conversation with him about problem solving? I think so.

And what did we learn from what the cop and I said about Lorenzo? Probably that drinking messes are just as common as the good times—no matter how infrequent we've been taught to perceive they are or try to tell each other they are.

And why did my son lose it? Because he didn't know any better? Maybe. It's true he jumped to judgment of Lorenzo, and that's not a nice or healthy perspective. But maybe his belief that everybody knows that it's a choice to drink responsibly is right on. And maybe his belief that everybody can do better when they know better—no matter their age, background or circumstance—is right on.

# Even With Eyes-Wide-Open, Seeing is Still a Choice

Remember at the beginning of this book when I compared figuring out our relationship with alcohol to discovering an alternate reality like the one in *The Matrix* movie? . . . remember the Morpheus quote inserted alongside the Contents Section? . . . the blue pills in the martini glass and red text on the cover? Obviously, I haven't been saying throughout this book that our awareness and use of alcohol is based on unknowingly being born into a machine-induced reality. However, the analogy I have been making is that we've been somewhat unknowingly living in an alcohol-induced reality since we were born. A reality that's based on acceptance and encouragement of a mind-altering and habit-forming substance whether we're drinking it or not. A reality that's based on a learned belief system of alcohol as a normal, frequent and controllable staple in adult life no matter how many drinking messes we make or see others make.

From a business and marketing perspective, the reality created by the alcohol companies is an absolutely-astoundingly-impressive accomplishment. Think about it. If you were to start a company today to sell a product whose most marketable reason for purchase (fun and relaxation) is the same reason for its most volatile side effects (regrets and apologies), you'd need an almost-blind-level of consumer buy-in to grow that business.

From a human-interest perspective, the reality that we encourage and defend about alcohol is equally impressive—but not always in a good way, so let's think for a minute about what this means too. Despite everyone experiencing mostly good times with alcohol, everyone also learns to be tolerant of the not-so-good times that alcohol can create. And even if the governments around the world were to require warning labels on alcohol packaging, or the nonprofits were to run more scare-tactic ads, I firmly believe no one would really pay attention to them anyway. So again, this just shows how powerful the influence of alcohol is in our reality.

Listen, in order to reduce the number and severity of accidents, arguments and addictions, and have any effect on the current omnipresent-level influence of alcohol, that parallel messaging would have to be as slick, positive and relatable as the alcohol messaging itself.

Which brings me back around to the question I asked a couple pages back: Is there anything bigger than *viral* marketing? I believe the answer is, *Yes.* And I believe the alcohol industry has achieved it. I call it *reality marketing.* And I define it as the three-spoke flywheel of paid advertising, word-of-mouth promotion, and free product placement in mainstream entertainment that self-generates an ever-growing momentum of sales.

So now that we can all agree to start recovering from being under the influence of the greatest sales strategy in the history of marketing, it's time to talk to my son about how this influence has contributed to his limiting beliefs and dismissive judgments about alcohol.

# THE CHOICE THAT'S TRULY YOURS

No Judgment

No Pressure

No Blame

Not a Poison

Not a Problem

Not a Conspiracy

Free Commerce

Free Will

Free To Be!

*. . . because the noblest pleasure*
*is the joy of understanding*

# No Judgment

My son and I are home alone in the kitchen.

He's shuffling school papers and texting on his phone while glancing at sports news on the muted TV. I decide now is the time to talk with him about his reaction to Lorenzo and about alcohol in general.

I'm clear about what I've learned while rethinking drinking, but I'm still a little nervous about how I'm going to say it to him. So I do what guys do when we need to talk about something important with each other: we mix the conversation into doing something mindless together. And since I don't have a view outside to sit and admire together, I decide to cook dinner while he's also in the kitchen doing his school things.

*Hey. Can you hear me while you're doing what you're doing?*

*Yeah. I'm just organizing my stuff for tomorrow. What's up?*

*Okay. I wanna circle-back and tie-up a few loose ends about alcohol and our recent experience with Lorenzo.*

My son stops organizing his school papers and looks up at me with an *Uh-oh* reaction on his face.

I give him a reassuring smile and head tilt.

*You didn't do anything wrong. But I do think that after you understand the whole story, you won't just think of him as an idiot. I want us to talk about a few key points while I cook dinner and you organize. Okay?*

*Okay. I'm in.*

*Great. Let's start with judgment. Mom and I have done a good job teaching you right from wrong. You're a good teenager who makes good choices, so we believe you're on your way to being a good man who will know what to pursue and how to achieve what you want while minimizing distractions throughout the rest of your life.*

He takes a deep breath and nods with his mouth pressed into an appreciating smile.

*However! I also want you to know is that the right and wrong you've been taught is our version . . . it's what Mom and I believe works to create a fulfilling and well-adjusted life. Not everybody chooses to live like we do.*

*Duh, Dad. I know everybody's different. But everybody knows that success comes from learning from our mistakes. So if Lorenzo's drinking is causing mistake after mistake, doesn't that make him not very bright?*

*I hear your point. But what I want you to know for sure is that everyone believes their reasoning is good for them. And when their results are repeatedly not good, when they persist without learning, it's usually because of some unresolved emotional thought or physical pain, which some people choose alcohol to comfort. So unless they're hurting someone else, we need to stay out of their stuff, and just see their stuff as a reminder to stay focused on achieving our stuff.*

*Okay, I hear you. I can let go of my judgment of what other people do and why they do it—unless they're hurting someone. But why would someone use alcohol to feel better rather than just solve their problem?*

*Good question.*

# No Pressure

The best way for me to answer your question about why some people repeatedly choose alcohol to dull a problem rather than solve a problem, even when it causes more problems, is to use you as an example.

*ME?! I solve my problems! Are you talking about the time I wrecked your car?!*

No. We both know you're resolving the car wreck problem by paying me back every week. What we're gonna talk about now is how people handle their stress and relieve the pressure they feel.

*Oh. Okay. But . . . huh?*

Stay with me, Player. I wanna walk you through this point by asking you a couple questions. When you have a really big sports achievement, do you celebrate with lots of pizza or cake or soda?

*No. I celebrate with my team. We turn up the music, dance and tell stories about the win. There might be food there, but none of us eats or drinks too much junk, because even though it tastes good we know it slows us down.*

Right. And when you mess up and get a bad grade on a school assignment, do you make yourself feel better by socializing 'til all hours of the night to get your mind off your mistake?

*Noooo. I figure out why I messed up. Then I find out from my teacher how to make it up and get my average back up. Then I socialize! But not too late into the night, because I don't like feeling tired the next day.*

Exactly. Last question in this example. When you're bored and wanna do something, but don't know what to do, do you plop in front of the TV and surf channels for hours and hours?

*No. I'd rather surf the internet and laugh at videos. But after a little while I get up from that. Bike ride. Run. Organize for tomorrow. I only plop for as long as I need to relax, then something'll come up that I wanna do.*

Definitely. Like I said a minute ago, you're a good teenager who makes good choices. And the reason for this is we've taught you to pay attention to how you feel when you're doing fun things, to understand mistakes are part of the goal process, to be patient that the answer will come when you don't know what *to do. And we've never used food to reinforce your fun, talk to gloss over a lesson, or screens to ease your boredom.*

*Whoa. I thought it was all me doing what I do.*

*It is all you. I'm sayin' Mom and I set you up with a good foundation for success, but at this point, YOU are the one choosing and achieving what you want. It's not that you don't feel stress, it's that you know how to handle it, because your parents and friends and activities are all aligned to support your feel-good pursuits. So if someone tries to pressure you into another slice of pizza or another hour at the party, it's easy for you to say 'no thanks' because you see how that choice would lead you away from the things that really make you feel good.*

*Ohhh. You're saying that Lorenzo's parents didn't teach him how to handle pressure. I follow you now! So it's his parents fault he drinks to feel better rather doing better?!*

*No. It's not his parents' fault. Lorenzo is a grown man who's been responsible for his choices since he was 18.*

*Oh! You're gonna tell me it's Lorenzo's fault! He's to blame, right?! Or maybe it's his wife's fault for getting mad and giving up on helping him to make better choices. It's gotta be somebody's fault.*

*Good question.*

# No Blame

$B$*efore I answer your question about blame, let's take a second to remind ourselves of the new per-spective we now have about judgment and pressure.*

*Yeah, I'm with ya . . . everybody's got their own good reason for doing what they do. And unless they're hurting someone, we need to just let them be, and make sure we're managing our own pressures to get the stuff we want.*

*Great. Thank you. Believe me, it's a much more enjoyable way to live.*

*I got it, Dad. Now tell me why someone would continue to drink if it creates bad results. Who's fault is it?*

*To answer your question, let's go back to how you told me you handle getting a low grade on a school project.*

*Yeah, I figure out why I messed up, then I ask my teacher how I can make it up.*

*Exactly. You ask your teacher for help. Or sometimes you ask my thoughts about whatever you're trying to fix.*

*Yes. Sooooo?*

*Listen, we don't really know what goes on between Lorenzo and Camilla next door. We had an experi-ence with them, and I'm using what I know about people and life and alcohol to hypothetically fill in the blanks in an effort to teach you an easier way to make sense of the world around you. But we don't really know all about Lorenzo and Camilla, and we no longer judge them for their circumstances anyway. Agreed?*

*Yes.*

*So, again, my guess about what we saw is the result of Lorenzo not asking Camilla for help with what-ever discomfort he may be feeling. And you know as well as I do that even when someone who cares is offering help, we usually can't hear them until we're ready to ask for it.*

*Yeah, I hear ya. I have kids in my classes who the teachers try to help with suggestions about how to pull their grades up, but those kids don't ask or listen because they think their grades are fine.*

*Now you're getting it.*

*Okay, I see now that it's not Camilla's fault or Lorenzo's parents' fault. I actually feel for them now. But why doesn't Lorenzo recognize that his drinking is causing pain and messes? How can that possibly be fine with him?*

*Just then, a huge reassuring smile comes over my face, and my son sees it.*

*What?*

*Now we're getting to the crux of this conversation about alcohol. The same way that a little alcohol alters an adult's thinking to feel a little easier, the more you drink, the more you wanna drink, and the less aware you become of how it's affecting your choices and your loved ones. It's way more powerful than chips and soda.*

*I promise I'm not being judgmental or blaming, Dad, but you're making alcohol sound like poison to me.*

*Good point. So let's talk a little more about what alcohol really is and what it does.*

# Not A Poison

---

Okay, Dad, so alcohol really is an unpredictable poison—right?

*I wouldn't say that. And the reason I don't believe it's poison is because most people's experience with alcohol matches the ads. It makes people feel relaxed and have fun, most people don't continue drinking to the point of losing their car or losing track of time or making a mess for their loved ones.*

Yeah, but alcohol messes do happen. And the risk of wanting to not drink responsibly is always there, right?

*Yes.*

Okay, then I'm going to think of it as poison.

At this point I realize my son may be defaulting back to judgment, and I've got to make sure he understands that what he chooses to believe is right for him does not mean that others are choosing wrong. I don't want him to miss out on good friendships and loving family experiences because he sees someone close to him drinking beer or even hears that someone got sick because they accidentally drank too much once or twice.

Listen, I agree with you that alcohol is unpredictable, but there's a better way to think of it than poison.

Okay. I'm listening.

The reason alcohol messes happen is just as much because of the people as it is the alcohol. That's why I don't want you to think of alcohol as poison or people as idiots. Neither the drink nor the drinker by themselves are to blame. It's the drinker's thoughts and feelings that mix with alcohol's relaxing effect that alters decision-making and causes the good times or the messes, and everything in between.

Ahhh. You're making another point about judgment?

Yes. And blame. Because remember, no one ever intends to drink and make a mess. But it's not a surprise because it does happen from time to time. And when it does, the drinker usually takes responsibility, and usually learns a lesson—but not always, for whatever reason—and then moves on.

---

*So you're saying again that I'll have an easier time in life if I let people live their way and do their thing?*

*Yes.*

*And I should also see alcohol for what it is? A relaxing drink for adults that may also cause unpredictable results?*

*Right ON, Son.*

*Okay. So if everyone knows how unpredictable alcohol is, why do so many relax and celebrate with it anyway?*

(Big proud smile)

*I'm so glad you asked.*

# Not A Problem

First of all, I wanna say that for you alcohol is not gonna be an automatic go-to for relaxation, fun or socializing, or become a problem.

*Yeah, because I'm not gonna drink!*

By the time you reach the legal drinking age and start deciding how much or how often to drink or not, I believe Mom and I will have guided you through enough practice in life to ever be tempted to believe alcohol is necessary or helpful.

*Oh, you mean like drinking rather than solving a problem?*

Yes. Or drinking just because it's what your friends are inviting you to do, after work, on the boat—whenever.

*Well, I'm pretty sure that alcohol is not for me. And I hear you that most people drink, and I'm fine with letting them be. But you haven't told me why so many people drink and some make mess after mess. And now I wanna know what other people's drinking has to do with my choice?*

It's the same answer to both questions: viral marketing.

*You mean like when people tell each other to use or buy something they saw advertised and tried?*

Yes. The thing about alcohol that makes so many people drink it is it actually does make you feel the way it looks in advertising and does what people say, so it makes sense that people recommend it to each other.

*Yeah, but what you said a minute ago is that alcohol also makes people want to drink more than they should and then risk losing control of themselves. So that makes alcohol sound to me like the problem.*

Yes, it's been my experience that sometimes people do wanna keep drinking more of it, and that's when there's a risk of it creating a problem. But I think that's why alcohol companies remind us to "Drink Responsibly" in their ads—because the effects of alcohol can be unpredictable when you drink too much or too often.

*Well, the ads are not clear. The reason I called Lorenzo an idiot is because I thought it was an easy choice to drink responsibly all the time. Now it seems like something is missing from the "Drink Responsibly" slogan.*

*I never paid much attention to the ads until you said that night Lorenzo must be an idiot because he doesn't follow the simple "Drink Responsibly" instructions. But since you said that, I started thinking about their ads.*

*So, is there something missing from the alcohol slogan? Something that would remind people that alcohol is not a solution to their problems? And maybe something about it being relaxing and fun but also easy to drink too much and cause yourself more problems?*

*Yes. I think so. And I've thought a lot about the few additional words that the alcohol companies could add to the bottom of their "Drink Responsibly" slogan. But if they never do it, I want you to know that I'm very proud of you for listening and understanding how all of this people and alcohol stuff we're talking about tonight could influence how you choose to live. I'm very comfortable that alcohol will not be a problem for you.*

*Got it, Daaaad! Now tell me the missing words you think would clarify the "Drink Responsibly" slogan!*

*Okay.*

# Not A Conspiracy

ere's the slightly more wordy slogan that I think would help people better understand the risks of alcohol without deterring them from the pleasures of drinking or slowing alcohol's huge viral marketing success:

**Drink Responsibly.**
**Alcohol is a mind-altering and habit-forming**
**substance that affects everyone differently.**

*I like it. Why do you think the alcohol ads don't include it? There's plenty of space on screens and billboards.*

(Laughing) *Because I think the alcohol companies think it's in their best interest to leave it the way it is.*

*What do you mean? What you said is clearer about what "Drink Responsibly" means, and still short to read.*

*I think if people were to see a clearer "Drink Responsibly" slogan, some may start talking about how slippery it is, and then maybe become more aware of themselves and their loved ones drinking too much or too often.*

*But isn't that the point the alcohol companies are making with their "Drink Responsibly" slogan?*

*Maybe. But I don't think people understand the current "Drink Responsibly" slogan as clearly as they could. It's been my experience while talking with friends and family that "Drink Responsibly" makes us believe that we're always in control and therefore always responsible for our results.*

*But you're not in control because you're saying as soon as you drink it, it's affecting your thinking.*

*Yes. And you'd think I would have figured out all of this sooner, because I turned 21 a long time ago. But I've been under the influence of fun alcohol advertising, the clever "Drink Responsibly" slogan, and innocent social encouragement from friends to believe I was in control of my alcohol thinking and responsible for my messes.*

*So it would be good for an expanded "Drink Responsibly" slogan to run . . . people might start talking about it like we have.*

*It would be good, but I think the chance of them expanding it is slim. So again, I'm glad we talked about it all tonight.*

*But why not, Dad? Why do you say it's not in the alcohol companies' best interest to clarify their slogan?*

*Because I think they think a clearer "Drink Responsibly" slogan might compromise their sales.*

*What?!*

*Think about it. You have alcohol ads showing all types of people with their product and smiles on their faces. You have TV, movies and music including alcohol in all types of social situations. You have people in real life getting together and usually matching the drinking experiences they see and hear in entertainment and ads. And when people do make a mess, the "Drink Responsibly" slogan reminds them it's their fault and to just control themselves next time. So if our talk tonight were to move the alcohol companies to expand their product slogan, some people might think twice before ordering another beer, which would reduce alcohol sales on a global scale.*

*Holy Shit, Dad! Alcohol isn't a poison . . . it's like an in-plain-sight conspiracy based on misleading advertising!*

*Oh boy. Alright. I see your point. But it's not a conspiracy. It's just free commerce.*

# Free Commerce

But Dad, how is this not a conspiracy?! It's almost like nobody really stands a chance to not become a drinker! Between the alcohol advertising . . . alcohol messages mixed into our TV, movies and music . . . and alcohol available and recommended everywhere we go, how can it all just be because of free commerce?!

Because the alcohol industry isn't intending harm. They're just selling a non-survival product that makes many people believe they need it to feel more relaxed and social. Because entertainers are just including alcohol to make their stories more relatable to people. And because there are laws in place to protect us from the possible harm of alcohol: it's not legal to drink alcohol under the age of 21 and it's not legal to drive while intoxicated.

But you're really smart, Dad, and you didn't realize how misleading all of it is until I called Lorenzo an idiot!

Thanks for that. Sometimes I can be smart about stuff.

We're both laughing now.

But yes, this is a new understanding for me. And it's an important one for navigating life. So that's why I'm sharing all of this with you. I think if my parents had known, they would have told me when I was your age too.

I hear you that the alcohol companies aren't intending harm. But by leaving the risks out of their product ads, isn't their half-truth advertising the reason their sales are so high and why everywhere we look it's for sale?

Sort of. The reason alcohol is for sale almost everywhere is a function of demand. If people didn't want it as much and as often as they do, it wouldn't be for sale almost everywhere we go.

Yeah, but people are buying their product because they don't completely understand how it affects them!

Again, sort of. I think the reason sales are so high is because alcohol delivers the feeling that's advertised, and people believe the viral messaging to each other: it's controllable fun, but messes happen, and it's our fault.

*Really?! You're saying that if people knew better about alcohol they wouldn't do better with their drinking?*

*I think some would think twice about how much and how often they drink and change their habits—and others wouldn't change a thing. Remember, when I said that everyone believes their reason for doing whatever they do is a good one?*

*Yeah, and not to judge them or blame them or feel pressure to drink because they're drinking. I got it.*

*Well, just like the alcohol companies simply advertising what's in their best interest to create more sales is called Free Commerce, people simply choosing alcohol for whatever reason they believe is in their best interest, without breaking the law, is called Free Will.*

# Free Will

Okay, Dad, what does free will have to do with people not choosing less alcohol if they knew better about it?

*Well . . . I think if an expanded "Drink Responsibly" slogan were to go viral and people started openly talking about it without judgment or blame, some would drink less. I think the viral conversations about what alcohol really is may make it easier on some trying to stop drinking. But, overall, I think most adults who are already in the habit of drinking wouldn't change at all.*

Wow. Really? Why do you think most people won't drink less, solve their stuff and make fewer messes?

*Remember, alcohol is a mind-altering and habit-forming substance—right?*

Yeah.

*And most people believe the "Drink Responsibly" slogan means everyone's in control of their good time and responsible if they make a mess—right?*

Yeah. We know those beliefs are not completely accurate now, but I hear ya.

*So, for the people who are already using the mind-altering part of alcohol for their normal socializing and relaxing—and still believe they're always in control, I think that it would take a lot of viral conversation about an expanded alcohol slogan to get most people to change.*

Geez. That really tells me how mind-altering and habit-forming alcohol is.

*Yes, the effects of alcohol really are very, very underestimated by most people. But we're just gonna let them freely choose to enjoy drinking to feel whatever they wanna feel—even if it leads to delaying some real solution, or annoying their loved ones, or whatever—right?*

Yes, I hear you about free will now.

*Good. Thank you. However! . . . the more I think about it, the more I believe that an expanded "Drink Responsibly" slogan would at least start to help upset wives like Camilla, and uninformed teenagers like you, to better understand alcohol good times, not-so-good times, and maybe avoid some awful messes.*

Yeah, this conversation we've had tonight definitely helps me understand alcohol better.

*Yes. And it was your free will to choose to listen and engage and consider another perspective about alcohol because of this talk, right? I didn't tell you it's bad, or not to drink, or people that do drink are wrong.*

*Yeah, I'm definitely gonna not judge people for drinking, or feel pressured to drink, because now I understand why it's so attractive to so many people, and how it can start as a social habit that could slip into causing some not-so-good times.*

*Very good, Son.*

*Thanks. So how do we get others to have this conversation?! This is really big, and useful for people to know!*

*Not sure. But I do agree with you that it would be awesome if everyone felt this free to be themselves, and free to let others do what they want with alcohol, and free to believe that drinking is not so necessary.*

# Free To Be!

**M**y son is lit-up. He's been sitting at the kitchen counter talking with me for the past half hour, but now he's up and pacing through the family room and kitchen. He's excited.

*There's gotta be something we can do to get people talking about this!*

*Yeah, I'm excited too. Our talk tonight does have me believing that since I was able to explain all of this to you, so you'd understand . . . maybe I can figure out how to do that next. And maybe the place to start this sort of parallel awareness campaign about alcohol would be with your age group.*

*Okaaaay . . . why?*

*Remember, I was your age once. And what I remember about me and all my friends is that during that time, we all wanted to do three things: drive a car, have sex, and drink alcohol.*

*Yeah, all of that is still true. Maybe not want to do, but definitely curious to do.*

*And, interestingly, as desirable and potentially dangerous as all three can be, the schools only help with what parents teach their kids at home by offering education for two of those three things.*

*Wow. That's true, Dad. I mean it isn't legal for kids to drink, but one ended up in an ambulance after he got really sick from drinking too much at a party one-night last year.*

*Yeah. Too many underage drinking stories like that. And too many like Lorenzo and Camilla.*

*Okay, Dad, you should figure out this Alcohol Ed stuff too. It's worthwhile for kids to know.*

*I agree. In the meantime, let's put a bow on tonight's conversation about alcohol.*

He finishes pacing and sits down at the kitchen counter. *Okay.*

*Basically what I've been saying to you tonight about judgment and blame for other people's choices is, those perspectives don't serve us. And even if others judge or blame or pressure you, when you know in your heart and mind that you're choosing what's best for you, then just let them be. I mean, try to have the conversation to help someone close to you understand your boundaries about alcohol or your inter- est in their well-being about their lack of alcohol boundaries. But if they disagree, sometimes we just have to walk away, wish them the best, and hope they just wanna talk with us about it later. Free To Be works both ways—okay?*

*I understand.*

*And here's the thing about the viral messaging for alcohol that is much slicker than when I was growing up . . . the celebrities endorsing alcohol in commercials and celebrities singing and acting with alcohol can be very tempting to wanna do what they do when we admire them.*

*Oh, you mean like that movie star I like in those glamorous gin commercials.*

*Yes, and that show we watch every Friday night with the Dad we admire grabbing a beer from the fridge when he gets home from work . . . and that awesome song we listen to at the gym about a fist full of whiskey.*

*Yeah, that song is the best!*

*I like all of those shows and movies and songs too. But the point I'm making is celebrities are also free to be. I think they're inadvertently teaching people how safe and normal alcohol is for everyone. But that doesn't mean they know better than you about how much, how often, or even if it's at all good for your life. Follow what I'm saying?*

*Yeah Dad, I hear you. But how did you figure all of this out.*

*I had to. I was Lorenzo for a long time. Making messes. Worrying loved ones. Stalled life.*

*What?!? YOU?!? But you haven't drank since you had 2 beers with Uncle Willy a while back.*

*Yeah, those 2 beers turned out to be a good reminder about the influence I was under. When I was much younger, I drank a lot-a lot, and it was all good, until it wasn't anymore. I had to straighten myself out for you and everyone I love, but mostly for me . . . so I just decided I didn't want to live that way anymore. No regrets and no blame. Alcohol just became too slippery for me.*

*Wow, Dad. I want to know what happened with you and alcohol.*

*I'll tell you about it sometime. But that's enough for tonight. Besides, dinner's ready and our favorite show is on TV!*

# ABOUT THE AUTHOR

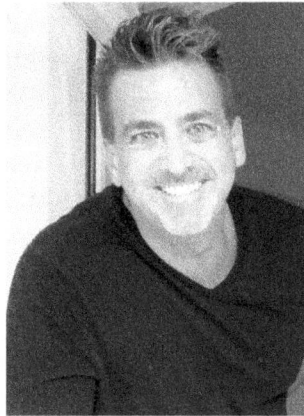

Craig Noble is a passionate pursuer of understanding. Usually, about professional and personal situations. Particularly, about people's motivation and results. Most recently, about how and why everyone is under the influence of alcohol. With an education that includes public school, state college and ivy league university; a career that ranges from large corporate environments to solo entrepreneurial callings; a personal life that spans super-achievers to confused-complainers; and a relationship with alcohol that runs from innocence to dependence to intelligence, Craig Noble brings a clever and fun perspective in *Rethinking Drinking* to help anyone start a new conversation about alcohol awareness. Craig can be reached through his website at www.rethinkingtheinfluence.com.